Rheumatic Diseases in Older Adults

Editors

JAMES D. KATZ
BRIAN WALITT

CLINICS IN
GERIATRIC MEDICINE

www.geriatric.theclinics.com

February 2017 • Volume 33 • Number 1

ELSEVIER

1600 John F. Kennedy Boulevard • Suite 1800 • Philadelphia, Pennsylvania, 19103-2899

http://www.theclinics.com

CLINICS IN GERIATRIC MEDICINE Volume 33, Number 1
February 2017 ISSN 0749–0690, ISBN-13: 978-0-323-49648-3

Editor: Jessica McCool
Developmental Editor: Colleen Viola

Clinics in Geriatric Medicine (ISSN 0749-0690) is published quarterly by Elsevier Inc., 360 Park Avenue South, New York, NY 10010-1710. Months of issue are February, May, August, and November. Business and Editorial Offices: 1600 John F. Kennedy Blvd., Suite 1800, Philadelphia, PA 191023-2899. Periodicals postage paid at New York, NY, and additional mailing offices. Subscription prices are $273.00 per year (US individuals), $590.00 per year (US institutions), $100.00 per year (US student/resident), $381.00 per year (Canadian individuals), $748.00 per year (Canadian institutions), $195.00 per year (Canadian student/resident), $402.00 per year (international individuals), $748.00 per year (international institutions), and $195.00 per year (international student/resident). Foreign air speed delivery is included in all *Clinics* subscription prices. All prices are subject to change without notice. POSTMASTER: Send address changes to *Clinics in Geriatric Medicine*, Elsevier Health Sciences Division, Subscription Customer Service, 3251 Riverport Lane, Maryland Heights, MO 63043. **Telephone: 1-800-654-2452 (U.S. and Canada); 314-447-8871 (outside U.S. and Canada). Fax: 314-447-8029. E-mail:** journalscustomerservice-usa@elsevier.com **(for print support)** or journalsonlinesupport-usa@elsevier.com **(for online support)**.

Reprints. For copies of 100 or more, of articles in this publication, please contact the Commercial Reprints Department, Elsevier Inc., 360 Park Avenue South, New York, New York 10010-1710. Tel.: 212-633-3874; Fax: 212-633-3820, E-mail: reprints@elsevier.com.

Clinics in Geriatric Medicine is covered in *MEDLINE/PubMed (Index Medicus)*, *EMBASE/Excerpta Medica, Current Contents/Clinical Medicine (CC/CM)*, and the *Cumulative Index to Nursing & Allied Health Literature*.

Contributors

EDITORS

JAMES D. KATZ, MD
Clinical Professor of Medicine, The George Washington University, Washington, DC; Rheumatology Fellowship Program Director, NIAMS/NIH, Bethesda, Maryland

BRIAN WALITT, MD, MPH
Medical Officer, NIDCR, NIH; Medical Officer, NINR, NIH, Bethesda, Maryland

AUTHORS

ANA T. ACEVEDO, MD
Rehabilitation Medicine Department, National Institutes of Health Clinical Center, Bethesda, Maryland

PALOMA ALEJANDRO, MD
Division of Rheumatology, MedStar Washington Hospital Center, Georgetown University Medical Center, Washington, DC

KATHARINE E. ALTER, MD
Rehabilitation Medicine Department, National Institutes of Health Clinical Center, Bethesda, Maryland

ALAN N. BAER, MD
Associate Professor, Division of Rheumatology, Department of Medicine, Johns Hopkins University School of Medicine, Baltimore, Maryland; National Institute of Dental and Craniofacial Research, National Institutes of Health, Bethesda, Maryland

ANN J. BIEHL, PharmD
Clinical Pharmacy Specialist, Department of Pharmacy, National Institutes of Health Clinical Center, Bethesda, Maryland

FLORINA CONSTANTINESCU, MD, MS, PhD
Division of Rheumatology, MedStar Washington Hospital Center, Georgetown University Medical Center, Washington, DC

ROBINDER J.S. DHILLON, MD, MBA
Fellow in Rheumatology, National Institute of Arthritis, and Musculoskeletal and Skin Diseases, National Institutes of Health, Bethesda, Maryland

HOSSAM EL-ZAWAWY, MD, MS
Assistant Professor, Charles E. Schmidt College of Medicine, Florida Atlantic University, Boca Raton; Staff, Department of Rheumatic and Immunologic Diseases, Cleveland Clinic Florida, Weston, Florida

MANDANA HASHEFI, MD, FACR
Assistant Professor of Medicine, Division of Rheumatology, The George Washington University, Washington, DC

SARFARAZ HASNI, MD
Director, Lupus Clinical Research Program, National Institute of Arthritis, and Musculoskeletal and Skin Diseases, National Institutes of Health, Bethesda, Maryland

ADRIENNE JACKSON, PT, PhD, MPA
Rehabilitation Medicine Department, National Institutes of Health Clinical Center, Bethesda, Maryland

JAMES D. KATZ, MD
Clinical Professor of Medicine, The George Washington University, Washington, DC; Rheumatology Fellowship Program Director, NIAMS/NIH, Bethesda, Maryland

LEWIS H. KULLER, MD, DrPH
Distinguished University Professor, Department of Epidemiology, University of Pittsburgh Graduate School of Public Health, Pittsburgh, Pennsylvania

RACHEL H. MACKEY, PhD, MPH, FAHA
Assistant Professor, Department of Epidemiology, University of Pittsburgh Graduate School of Public Health, University of Pittsburgh, Pittsburgh, Pennsylvania

UNA E. MAKRIS, MD, MSc
Assistant Professor, Division of Rheumatic Diseases, Department of Internal Medicine, UT Southwestern Medical Center, VA North Texas Health Care System, Dallas, Texas

BRIAN F. MANDELL, MD, PhD, FACR
Professor and Chairman of Academic Medicine, Department of Rheumatic and Immunologic Disease, Cleveland Clinic Lerner College of Medicine, Cleveland, Ohio

DEVYANI MISRA, MD, MSc
Assistant Professor, Section of Clinical Epidemiology, Department of Medicine, Boston University School of Medicine, Boston, Massachusetts

LARRY W. MORELAND, MD
Chief, Division of Rheumatology and Clinical Immunology, University of Pittsburgh School of Medicine, Pittsburgh, Pennsylvania

NORA TAYLOR, MD, FACR
Assistant Professor of Medicine, Division of Rheumatology, The George Washington University, Washington, DC

BRIAN WALITT, MD, MPH
Medical Officer, NIDCR, NIH; Medical Officer, NINR, NIH, Bethesda, Maryland

RAYMOND YUNG, MD, MB, ChB
Professor and Chief, Division of Geriatric and Palliative Medicine, Department of Internal Medicine, VA Ann Arbor Health System, University of Michigan, Ann Arbor, Michigan

Contents

> Providing safe and effective pharmacotherapy to the geriatric patients with rheumatological disorders is an ongoing struggle for the rheumatologist and geriatrician alike. Cohesive communication and partnership can improve the care of these patients and subvert adverse outcomes. Disease-modifying antirheumatic drugs, including methotrexate, hydroxy-chloroquine, sulfasalazine, and leflunomide, and the newest oral agent for treatment of rheumatoid arthritis, tofacitinib, have distinctive monitoring and adverse effect profiles. This article provides the general practitioner or geriatrician with clinically relevant pearls regarding the use of these interventions in older patients.

> Sarcopenia represents a loss of muscle strength and mass in older individuals. Sarcopenia in the elderly has now become a major focus of research and public policy debate due to its impact on morbidity, mortality, and health care expenditure. Despite its clinical importance, sarcopenia remains under-recognized and poorly managed in routine clinical practice. This is, in part, due to a lack of available diagnostic testing and uniform diagnostic criteria. The management of sarcopenia is primarily focused on physical therapy for muscle strengthening and gait training. There are no pharmacologic agents for the treatment of sarcopenia.

> Osteoporosis in the elderly population is common. It results in more than 1.5 million fractures per year in the United States. The goal of managing osteoporosis is to prevent fractures. In men, osteoporosis is underrecognized and undertreated. More men than women die every year as a consequence of hip fractures. A review of diagnosis and treatment of osteoporosis is described in this article. Bisphosphonates are the first-line treatment for men and women. In the past several years, advances in bone biology have resulted in major therapeutic advances.

> Symptomatic knee osteoarthritis is a common complaint of many elderly patients in primary care offices. For those unable or unwilling to undergo

knee replacement, the primary practitioners' understanding of the strengths and weaknesses of the available treatment modalities for pain relief is critical to successful in-office counseling and expectation management. Treatment requires a multimodal approach of nonpharmacologic and pharmacologic therapies to achieve a maximal clinical benefit. The focus of this review is on the nonsurgical options for treatment of knee osteoarthritis in patients aged 65 and older.

Musculoskeletal problems are the most frequently reported complaints among older adults living in the community. The impact of the aging process on skeletal muscles and joints can have a profound effect on the ability of individuals with and without disabilities to function. This article reviews the rehabilitation medicine approach to the evaluation of older adults with regional rheumatic disorders, and the rehabilitation medicine considerations for clinical interventions. Future research considerations are encouraged in order to gain a greater understanding of the subject matter and its impact on the provision of care and patients' quality of life.

A variety of conditions mimicking rheumatologic syndromes may be associated with an underlying malignancy. Therefore, distinguishing these syndromes from more common, nonparaneoplastic rheumatologic conditions can be perplexing. Some autoimmune conditions and the medications used for their management can be associated with increased future risk of malignancy. Some cancers can directly involve the musculoskeletal structures, whereas others present with systemic manifestations at sites away from the tumor and its metastases. Better awareness and timely recognition of these associations may lead to earlier cancer detection and hopefully better long-term survival.

Dry eye and dry mouth symptoms are each reported by up to 30% of persons more than 65 years of age, particularly in women. Medication side effects are the most common contributing factors. The evaluation of these symptoms requires measures of ocular and oral dryness. Sjögren syndrome is the prototypic disease associated with dryness of the eyes and mouth and predominantly affects women in their perimenopausal and postmenopausal years. In addition to topical treatment of the mucosal dryness, patients with Sjögren syndrome may require treatment with systemic immunomodulatory and immunosuppressive agents to manage a variety of extraglandular manifestations.

Evidence suggests the greater than 1.5 increased risk of cardiovascular disease (CVD) in rheumatoid arthritis (RA) is related to an accelerated burden of subclinical atherosclerosis that develops before the diagnosis of RA. Dyslipidemia in RA is better quantified by lipoproteins and apolipoproteins than cholesterol levels. Current risk factors likely underestimate CVD risk partly by underestimating prior risk factor levels. To reduce CVD risk in RA, control disease activity and aggressively treat CVD risk factors. Some of the two-fold higher risk of heart failure and total mortality in RA may be due to myocardial disease caused by inflammation.

The incidence and prevalence of rheumatologic conditions are increasing and the rheumatology workforce must be aware of aging-specific issues. This article reviews specific barriers to understanding the biology of aging and aging-related mechanisms that may underlie development of rheumatologic diseases in older adults. It summarizes gaps in the assessment, outcomes measurement, and treatment of these diseases in this unique population. It also highlights potential solutions to these barriers and suggests possible ways to bridge the gap, from a research and education standpoint, so that clinicians can be better prepared to effectively manage older adults with rheumatologic conditions.

The prevalence of gout increases with age. Once serum concentration of urate exceeds the saturation/solubility point, it deposits in and around the joints. Clinical presentation in the elderly often has "atypical" features and is challenging to diagnose. Treatment depends on the stage of the disease and the patient's health status and comorbidities. Elderly patients often have several confounding issues; thus, treatment decisions can be complicated and therapeutic options limited. To prevent the recurrence of gout attacks, serum concentration of urate should be maintained well below the saturation threshold of 6.8 mg/dL, leading to dissolution of urate deposits and prevent recurrence.

CLINICS IN GERIATRIC MEDICINE

THE CLINICS ARE AVAILABLE ONLINE!
Access your subscription at:
www.theclinics.com

Preface

Rheumatic Diseases in Older Adults

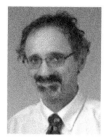 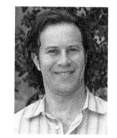

James D. Katz, MD   Brian Walitt, MD, MPH
Editors

We are pleased to present this special issue of *Clinics in Geriatric Medicine* that is devoted to Rheumatic Diseases in Older Adults. To this end, we have assembled a broad range of expertise in order to highlight the latest diagnostic and therapeutic information in the field. Our agenda has not been to re-invent a general overview of geriatric rheumatology but rather to hone in on pragmatic as well as up-and-coming musculoskeletal issues facing gerontologists.

The choice of contributors herein reflects our bias that rheumatologists and other academicians who are involved in the rheumatologic aspects of aging are well suited to address the impact of musculoskeletal issues affecting function and mobility. Hence, within these pages, you will find not only clinical pearls helping the practitioner to navigate underappreciated aspects of pharmacotherapeutics but also, for example, a nuanced rheumatologic perspective on sarcopenia.

As Guest Editors, we have encouraged broad thinking among our authorship. Our contributors have been tasked not to lose sight of the principle of aging in place while aiming to drive forward thoughtful discussion within the gerontology community.[1] Therefore, interspersed among these pages may be found both philosophical perspectives and potential policy-shaping research agendas. As such, we hope this issue serves to further the study of quality of life in an aging demographic. Finally, we hope that by invoking rheumatologic insight, we have broadened the clinical horizon sufficiently so as to challenge the perspectives of educators, practitioners, and academicians alike. Perhaps now is the time to move our respective disciplines

Clin Geriatr Med 33 (2017) ix–x
http://dx.doi.org/10.1016/j.cger.2016.10.001
0749-0690/17/© 2016 Published by Elsevier Inc.

geriatric.theclinics.com

forward from "OsteoRheumatology"[2] to what might be more aptly termed, "GerontoRheumatology."

James D. Katz, MD
NIAMS/NIH

Brian Walitt, MD, MPH
NIDCR
NINR, NIH

E-mail addresses:
James.katz@nih.gov (J.D. Katz)
brian.walitt@nih.gov (B. Walitt)

REFERENCES

1. Morley JE. Aging successfully: the key to aging in place. J Am Med Dir Assoc 2015;16(12):1005–7.
2. Favero M, Giusti A, Geusens P, et al. OsteoRheumatology: a new discipline? RMD Open 2015;1(Suppl 1):e000083.

Pharmacotherapy Pearls for the Geriatrician

Focus on Oral Disease-Modifying Antirheumatic Drugs Including Newer Agents

Ann J. Biehl, PharmD[a],*, James D. Katz, MD[b]

KEYWORDS

- Geriatrics • DMARDs • Rheumatology • Tofacitinib

KEY POINTS

- Older rheumatology patients are at increased risk for therapeutic misadventure due to age-related pharmacokinetic and pharmacodynamic changes, polypharmacy, impaired health literacy secondary to decreased cognition, and provider age bias.
- Geriatricians, working in partnership with rheumatologists and other members of the allied health care team, can most effectively minimize the risk for medication-related adverse events in older patients.
- Familiarity with dosing, monitoring, medication interactions, potential for commonly encountered adverse effects and amelioration strategies can improve the safety of disease-modifying antirheumatic drugs and tofacitinib in the older rheumatology patient.

INTRODUCTION

Providing safe and effective pharmacotherapy to the geriatric patient population is an ongoing struggle for health care providers. The incidence of chronic health conditions such as rheumatological disorders increases with advancing age.[1] Data from the annual 2014 National Health Interview Survey indicate that 47.4% of adults ages 65 to 74 carry a diagnosis of arthritis. This estimate rises to 50.9% in adults ages 75 years and greater.[1] It is estimated that rheumatoid arthritis affects 0.5% to 1% of the adult population in developed countries. In the United States, this translates to approximately 1.3 million adults, with an increasing prevalence with older age.[2]

Disclosure Statement: This work was supported by the Intramural Program of the National Institute of Arthritis and Musculoskeletal and Skin Diseases (NIAMS) of the National Institutes of Health (NIH).

[a] Department of Pharmacy, National Institutes of Health Clinical Center, 10 Center Drive, Room 1C240, Bethesda, MD 20892-1196, USA; [b] National Institutes of Arthritis and Musculoskeletal and Skin Diseases, National Institutes of Health, 6N-216F, Building 10, 9000 Rockville Pike, Bethesda, MD 20892, USA
* Corresponding author.
E-mail address: ann.biehl@nih.gov

Oral disease-modifying antirheumatic drugs (DMARDs) can ameliorate some auto-immune diseases and improve morbidity and mortality. The geriatrician should be aware of specific issues associated with the use of oral DMARDs in aging patients. For example, newer agents such as Janus kinase (JAK) inhibitors for treatment of rheumatoid arthritis and urate transporter inhibitors for treatment of gout require special consideration before their use in the elderly patient.

Older patients are at increased risk for adverse drug reactions. Despite that people older than the age of 65 years make up 14% of the US population, Budnitz and colleagues[3] found that patients older than 65 years of age accounted for 25% of emergency room visits for adverse drug reactions. Such therapeutic misadventures in geriatric patients can be due to age-related changes in pharmacokinetics and pharmacodynamics, polypharmacy contributing to increased risk of clinically significant drug-drug interactions, and alterations in cognitive faculties that impair health literacy and therapeutic adherence.[4–9] These problems are likely compounded by age bias, manifesting as a reluctance to aggressively treat older patients, as well as economic barriers.[10,11] In addition to the physiologic and social factors contributing to the risk of adverse drug events in the elderly, management of rheumatologic conditions carries special risk due to rapidly evolving use of novel therapeutic agents and limited data supporting their use in geriatric patients.

This review article provides an update regarding commonly used oral DMARDs for the treatment of inflammatory arthritis, including methotrexate, hydroxychloroquine (HCQ), sulfasalazine (SSZ), and leflunomide, as well as serves to review pertinent information regarding the newest oral anti rheumatic agent, tofacitinib. Special considerations regarding the role of the developing field of pharmacogenetics, immunization practices for the older rheumatology patient and areas of future research are also discussed. Although nonsteroidal anti-inflammatories, prednisone, and injectable biologic agents are commonly used in the management of inflammatory arthritis, these are outside the scope of this article.

AGE-RELATED CHANGES IN DRUG METABOLISM

Geriatric patients experience physiologic changes at every step of the pharmacokinetic process. However, the general lack of inclusion of older adults in clinical trials and drug-specific pharmacokinetic studies has been a great obstacle in the understanding of the age-related changes on pharmacokinetic properties of particular medications. Physiologic pharmacokinetic changes in elderly patients have been outlined extensively in prior review articles.[6,8] The most clinically significant pharmacokinetic alteration in this population is a decline in renal function that inhibits excretion of metabolites. Many commonly used antirheumatic medications require monitoring of renal function, including methotrexate.

Aging patients also experience changes in pharmacodynamic processes or in the magnitude of end organ effects. Mechanistically, these changes can occur at a receptor level or secondary to the age-related blunting of other compensatory systems.[6] Older patients are more sensitive to the effects of a multitude of medications, including antihypertensives such as beta-blockers, diuretics, anticoagulants, antihyperglycemics, and NSAIDs. For example, due to a decrease of cell density of bone marrow, elderly patients may be more sensitive to the development of anemia during methotrexate therapy. Therefore, selecting more conservative initial doses and more gradual increases in dose titration is a common clinical strategy for managing antirheumatic therapy in older individuals.[6]

POLYPHARMACY

Polypharmacy has been defined in many ways in modern medicine. Some definitions focus on a set number of medications, ranging from 2 to 10 or more, medications, whereas others define polypharmacy as any medication that is not clinically appropriate or indicated.[9,12–14] Consequences to polypharmacy include the risk for clinically significant drug-drug interactions, adverse drug reactions, and nonadherence due to complicated drug regimens.[9]

Age is a commonly cited risk factor for polypharmacy.[12] Geriatric patients with polypharmacy are at special risk for cognitive impairment, falls, incontinence, and poor nutritional status.[9] Not surprisingly, older rheumatoid arthritis patients are at risk because of complex medical regimens. Treharne and colleagues[15] found that the total number of medications for rheumatoid arthritis patients was predicted by older age and longer duration of rheumatoid arthritis. In addition, the total number of comorbidities contributed to this relationship. The same is true for hospitalized patients. A 2001 study of hospitalized subjects with rheumatic diseases found similar results, with older subjects having higher likelihood of meeting the study's definition of polypharmacy compared with younger subjects.[16]

HEALTH LITERACY

Health literacy, defined as an individual's overall capacity to obtain, process, and understand basic health information and services needed to make appropriate health decisions, is another area in which age-related changes may have an impact.[17] In 2014, Wong and colleagues[18] noted that up to one-third of patients who are prescribed common rheumatology medications followed dosing instructions incorrectly, underscoring the importance of health literacy in contributing to safe and effective care. Several studies have found a relationship between older age and reduced health literacy; however, this relationship can be confounded by educational level and commonly encountered age-related changes affecting functional status, such as visual impairment.[4,19–21] An observational cohort study by Barton and colleagues[22] identified age older than 55 years as a risk factor for poor knowledge of methotrexate in a diverse urban rheumatology clinic population in California.

AGE BIAS

Older patients may face yet another challenge in receiving safe and effective treatment of rheumatological disorders in the form of age bias, or disparities in the prescription of treatment by doctors based on patient age.[23,24] In a 2010 choice-based conjoint analysis, Kievit and colleagues[10] showed that among 135 rheumatologists, younger patient age ranked second behind more severe disease activity (as defined by the disease activity [DAS] score) in dictating the decision to escalate treatment of rheumatoid arthritis. The reluctance to escalate therapy due to concerns about comorbidities, adverse drug reactions, and polypharmacy may result in older patients not receiving appropriate interventions, despite that elderly patients demonstrate a similar responsiveness to standard therapies when compared with younger patients.[11,25]

Due to these complexities, geriatricians, working in partnership with rheumatologists and other members of the allied health care team, can most effectively minimize the risk for therapeutic misadventure.

METHOTREXATE

Methotrexate was first found to be efficacious in the management of inflammatory arthritis in the 1950s but did not receive Food and Drug Administration (FDA) approval for the treatment of rheumatoid arthritis until 1988.[26,27] Since that time, low-dose methotrexate has become one of the most commonly used DMARDs for treating rheumatoid arthritis in adult patients of all ages.[28–31]

Methotrexate inhibits purine and pyrimidine synthesis through inhibition of dihydrofolate reductase, which confers activity in antineoplastic indications, as well as dictates certain toxicities. However, its antiinflammatory mechanism of action likely differs from its antimetabolite effect in that it inhibits aminoimidazole-carboxamido ribonucleotide (AICAR) transformylase, which initiates a signaling cascade that increases adenosine release and ultimately decreases synthesis of proinflammatory cytokines, including tumor necrosis factor alpha, interleukin (IL)-6, and interferon-gamma, as well as increases production of antiinflammatory cytokines such as IL-10.[32,33]

Once weekly methotrexate can be administered orally or via subcutaneous or intramuscular injection. From a practical standpoint, intramuscular injection is used less frequently than the other administration options. The bioavailability of oral methotrexate decreases with increasing dose.[34] A 2014 randomized cross-over study by Schiff and colleagues[35] showed that systemic exposure of oral methotrexate plateaued at doses equal to, or greater than, 15 mg weekly, whereas subcutaneous administration at the same doses resulted in linear increases in systemic exposure. Therefore, changing to subcutaneous injection in the setting of higher doses will improve bioavailability.[35] Methotrexate is converted in the liver to active metabolites which are eliminated primarily via renal excretion and therefore may accumulate in the setting of impaired renal function.[36]

Patients are more likely to discontinue methotrexate secondary to intolerance as opposed to lack of efficacy.[37] Adverse effects of weekly methotrexate include gastrointestinal intolerance, including nausea, vomiting, abdominal pain, and stomatitis; elevation of hepatic enzymes; photosensitivity; alopecia; pulmonary side effects, including pneumonitis; and hematologic abnormalities, including megaloblastic anemia, leukopenia, thrombocytopenia, and pancytopenia.[7,38] It is imperative to note that the incidence of many methotrexate-induced adverse effects can be related to impaired renal function and, therefore, it is prudent to routinely evaluate renal function in geriatric patients on such therapy.[30,39]

Folic acid supplementation may ameliorate some of the folate-pathway–dependent adverse effects related to low-dose methotrexate therapy without significant impact on treatment efficacy. A 2013 Cochrane review that included 6 randomized, double-blind, placebo-controlled trials examining the impact of folic or folinic acid supplementation on methotrexate therapy for rheumatoid arthritis concluded that such supplementation reduced the discontinuation rate of methotrexate therapy for any reason, as well as reduced the incidence of abnormal transaminase development.[40] Although not statistically significant, reductions in the incidence of gastrointestinal adverse effects, including stomatitis, were also noted. The impact of folic or folinic acid supplementation on hematologic side effects could not be adequately assessed due to the infrequent rate of hematologic sequelae.[40]

The optimal dose of folic acid has yet to be elucidated. In a 2015 randomized controlled trial, Dhir and colleagues[41] showed that there was no additional benefit with regard to tolerability or treatment-blunting effects for a dose of 30 mg/week of folic acid compared with the lower dose of 10 mg/week of folic acid. Dosing schemes vary greatly, with administration of 1 mg/day of folic acid being common practice.[42]

Methotrexate's inhibition of the folate pathway also contributes to medication interactions with other folic acid antagonists. In a 2010 review of 67 articles addressing medication interactions with low-dose methotrexate, Bourre-Tessier and Haraoui[43] noted that the commonly prescribed folate antagonist trimethoprim-sulfamethoxazole (TMP-SMX) was identified as a major risk factor in the development of cytopenias in 1 observational study and 17 case reports. In these cases, TMP-SMX was most commonly prescribed as a treatment of cystitis with most cases of pancytopenia identified between 2 days and 2 weeks of starting TMP-SMX therapy. In contradistinction, there were no reported cases of bone marrow suppression identified with prophylactic TMP-SMX dosed 3 times/week for pneumocystis prevention.

Clinical pearls: methotrexate

- Monitor renal function; dose adjust accordingly.
- Folic acid supplementation can improve tolerability with minimal effects on efficacy.
- Avoid use of concomitant folate antagonists, including TMP-SMX when dosed daily.

HYDROXYCHLOROQUINE

HCQ is another commonly used DMARD for management of a multitude of rheumatological disorders. HCQ carries FDA approval for treatment of rheumatoid arthritis and systemic lupus erythematosus (SLE). Treatment with HCQ was found to be an independent determinant of remission in rheumatoid arthritis in a multicenter cross-sectional study. HCQ has exhibited synergistic effects in improving disease activity when used in combination with other DMARDs, including methotrexate and SSZ.[44,45] Therapy with HCQ has demonstrated a beneficial effect in morbidity and mortality outcomes in SLE patients.[46,47]

HCQ is generally regarded as well-tolerated, with gastrointestinal distress being the most common adverse effect. Skin hyperpigmentation is also a known side effect of long-term HCQ therapy. There are case reports in the literature of HCQ-induced blue-black dyschromia being clinically misinterpreted as elder abuse. These cases were resolved after a thorough history or, in some cases, a skin biopsy.[48,49]

HCQ also has the potential to cause the serious side effect of irreversible retinal toxicity. HCQ-induced retinopathy was initially thought to be quite rare; however, this assessment was based on studies of short duration and diagnoses of fairly advanced retinopathy.[50] Current literature indicates that HCQ-induced retinopathy is more common than originally estimated.[51] This is most likely due to improved detection methods and frequency of screening. A 2014 retrospective case-control study by Melles and Marmor[51] reviewed more than 2300 patient records of HCQ users with at least 5 years of treatment duration in a large integrated health organization of 3.4 million overall members. Data from this study yielded an overall prevalence of HCQ-related retinopathy of 7.5%, with occurrence of retinopathy varying with dose and duration of treatment.

In addition to duration of use, the investigators identified the following as risk factors for the development of retinopathy: total daily dose of HCQ; presence of kidney disease as defined by glomerular filtration rate of less than 60 mL/minute or presence of stage 3, 4, or 5 kidney disease on their problem list; and concurrent tamoxifen use. Age itself was not identified as a risk factor.

Historically, the upper limit of dosing for HCQ to avoid toxicity was thought to be 6.5 mg HCQ/kg based on ideal body weight. However, Melles and colleagues concluded that actual body weight was a better predictor of toxicity.[51] The investigators concluded that 6.5 mg/kg ideal body weight corresponded to 5.0 mg/kg actual body weight and recommended using 5.0 mg/kg of real body weight in assessing appropriate HCQ dosing in the future. Patients exceeding 5.0 mg/kg HCQ exhibited a 10% risk of retinal toxicity within 10 years of HCQ use and an almost 40% risk after 20 years of treatment.

Routine ophthalmic HCQ retinopathy screening is recommended in patients with an expected extended duration of therapy and should include an initial assessment at baseline followed by annual screening with 10-2 visual fields. This should include more sensitive, objective tests, including spectral domain optical coherence tomography or multifocal electroretinogram, starting no later than after 5 years of use.[52]

Recently, attention has turned to using principles of therapeutic drug monitoring to HCQ through the use of high performance liquid chromatography; however, there is profound variability in the resultant whole blood levels with contributing factors to this observation not fully defined.[53–55] Although these levels may be used to assess adherence, their ability to predict the potential for development of retinal toxicity has not yet been established.[56] Furthermore, these levels are not widely commercially available and, therefore, are not readily accessible to the health care provider.

Clinical pearls: HCQ

- Estimates of the prevalence of retinal toxicity are more frequent than historically appreciated.
- Judicious dosing to avoid toxicity should be practiced using a 5.0 mg/kg actual body weight cut-off.
- Routine ophthalmology examinations are recommended to screen for the development of retinal toxicity.

SULFASALAZINE

SSZ has a prominent role in the treatment of inflammatory arthritis in patients of all ages. Indeed, SSZ enjoys international popularity.[57] In part, this popularity may relate to both the cost-effectiveness of this agent and the reduced risk for infection relative to newer therapies.[58,59] In the United States, SSZ ranks among the top four DMARDs used for the treatment of rheumatoid arthritis.[60,61]

SSZ is composed of sulfapyridine and 5-aminosalicylic acid. It is thought that the antiarthritic activity of this compound is conferred by the sulfapyridine moiety. Genetic polymorphisms may play a role in the efficacy of the drug as well as the propensity for adverse effects. In particular, a prolonged half-life of the sulfapyridine metabolite of SSZ may be seen in slow acetylators. However, the clinical importance of this has yet to be fully adjudicated.[62]

Although it may be used alone, triple therapy, including SSZ, methotrexate, and HCQ, is an established therapeutic regimen. On longitudinal follow-up, SSZ is the most commonly discontinued drug in this regimen secondary to adverse effects.[63]

Owing to the possibility of SSZ causing hemolytic anemia, screening patients for glucose-6-phosphate dehydrogenase (G-6-PD) deficiency before initiating the drug may be considered.[64] Another adverse bone marrow effect may occur due to inhibition of intracellular folate metabolism thereby contributing to megaloblastic anemia.

Gastrointestinal complaints are common with initiation of SSZ and are dose-related. Gastrointestinal issues are usually mild in nature and resolve with continuation or dose reduction of SSZ.[65] The enteric-coated formulation may be better tolerated than the regular release formulation of SSZ.[66]

A noteworthy syndrome of fever, rash, and abnormal liver indices secondary to SSZ therapy may occur. In the presence of eosinophilia, this reaction is termed drug rash with eosinophilia and systemic symptoms (DRESS).[67] It is possible that this reaction is a forme fruste of the hemophagocytic syndrome and, hence, justifies avoiding further use of the agent.[68]

A rare adverse effect of SSA is crystalluria and subsequent anuric renal failure.[69] Therefore, vigilance toward maintaining adequate hydration is prudent in older individuals treated with SSZ.

Finally, azoospermia is a well-documented potential adverse effect of SSZ that may, in turn, impact fertility.[70]

Clinical pearls: SSZ

- SSZ-mediated inhibition of intracellular folate metabolism may contribute to the development of megaloblastic anemia.
- Gastrointestinal side effects are common on treatment initiation and usually dose-related.
- Crystalluria is a rare adverse effect. Patients should maintain adequate hydration.

LEFLUNOMIDE

Leflunomide is an isoxazole derivate that inhibits the pyrimidine pathway and seems to modulate T-cell immunology by shifting the T-helper (Th)1/Th2 balance.[71] Consequently, it has successfully been used in the treatment of various inflammatory arthritides. Moreover, leflunomide seems to enjoy a similar safety profile regardless of the age of the patient.[72] That being said, the safe prescribing of this agent relies on monitoring not only the blood count and liver function but also blood pressure. Unfortunately, the embryotoxicity and teratogenicity of this agent renders it less appealing for use during the childbearing years. More recent data suggest that among the DMARDs, patients on leflunomide may be more prone to unintentional weight loss, which could be of concern in older patients who are frail.[73] In this regard, genetic polymorphisms of CYP2C9 and CYP1A2 may be predictive of therapy cessation due to side effects, including weight loss.[74,75]

Due to low hepatic clearance and enterohepatic recycling, the pharmacokinetic profile of leflunomide is notable for a long elimination half-life of approximately 2 weeks.[76] In the setting of severe toxicity or other condition necessitating rapid withdrawal, cholestyramine can be used to bind the active metabolite of leflunomide in the intestine and interrupt enterohepatic or entero-entero recycling, thus reducing the half-life to 1 to 2 days.[76–79]

Clinical pearls: leflunomide

- The safety and adherence profiles of leflunomide do not change with increasing patient age.
- Regardless of this, hypertension and unintentional weight loss are 2 adverse effects related to leflunomide therapy that may be of particular concern in older patients.
- In the clinical scenarios in which rapid withdrawal of leflunomide is indicated, a cholestyramine washout can be implemented to decrease the half-life of the active metabolite.

TOFACITINIB

Tofacitinib, a targeted synthetic DMARD, is the newest oral agent in the armamentarium of treatment of rheumatoid arthritis. Tofacitinib has a novel mechanism of action of JAK inhibition. JAK inhibition results in decreased signaling of proinflammatory cytokines that drive lymphocyte activation and function.[80]

Approved by the FDA in 2012, tofacitinib has been studied with and without background methotrexate and has proved efficacious in patients with refractory rheumatoid arthritis.[81–84] The full potential of tofacitinib remains unknown in the management of autoimmune disorders. Trials are currently underway studying the agent's effects in management of disease states, including juvenile idiopathic arthritis, SLE, psoriatic arthritis, and ankylosing spondylitis (available at: clinical trials.gov). The effects of tofacitinib have also been explored in areas outside of rheumatology, including prevention of organ transplant rejection, with promising results.[85–87]

Tofacitinib is FDA-approved for daily dosing at 5 mg twice daily or with the extended release formulation at 11 mg once daily. Tofacitinib is metabolized via CYP 450 3A4 and 2C19, and the potential for clinically significant medication interactions exist with strong inhibitors of these enzymes, as well as dual moderate inhibitors of both enzymes.[88]

As with other DMARDs, increased risk of infection is a concern with tofacitinib. A 2014 study examining pooled data from 2 long-term safety studies following subjects on tofacitinib 5 mg twice daily or 10 mg twice daily (with or without background DMARDs) for up to 60 months found an overall risk of serious infection of 4.5% (3.1 events/100 patient years). This event rate was dose related, with more serious infections recorded in the 10 mg twice a day group.[89] Additional independent predictors associated with increased risk of serious infections include age older than 65 years, corticosteroid doses greater than 7.5 mg daily of prednisone (or equivalent), and presence of diabetes. Opportunistic infections, including tuberculosis and herpes zoster, were also observed; therefore, screening for tuberculosis is recommended before therapy initiation.[31,89] A 2015 meta-analysis concluded that overall serious infection rates with tofacitinib were comparable to biologic agents but this conclusion is limited by a paucity of direct comparator trials.[90]

In long-term extension studies, the risk of herpes zoster in patients on tofacitinib seemed to be elevated beyond the frequency reported in the literature for patients receiving alternative DMARD or biologic agents.[89] Incidence rates of herpes zoster in Asian patients also seem to be higher, with the highest rates of herpes zoster occurring in Japanese and Korean patients.[91] The investigators concluded that preventative strategies for herpes zoster should be developed for patients with rheumatoid arthritis. The administration of herpes zoster vaccine is conditionally recommended in patients with rheumatoid arthritis older than age 50 years and before initiation with biologic therapy or tofacitinib.[31] Despite this recommendation, vaccination against herpes zoster is woefully underutilized in patients with rheumatoid arthritis and, hence, the primary care provider may have a profound impact in this area.[92]

In addition to considering vaccination against herpes zoster in appropriate patients before commencing tofacitinib therapy, the primary care provider plays an integral role in ensuring the appropriate administration of other vaccinations including pneumococcal polysaccharide vaccine (PPSV-23), as well as the annual influenza vaccine in patients who are currently receiving or considering initiation with tofacitinib therapy. Winthrop and colleagues[93] illustrated a diminished responsiveness to PPSV-23 in subjects commencing tofacitinib therapy at a dose of 10 mg twice daily. Response was further diminished in subjects on concomitant methotrexate. However, response to annual influenza vaccination was unaltered in subjects receiving tofacitinib with or without methotrexate. In current users, a 2-week holiday from tofacitinib around the time of vaccination did not appreciably improve immunogenicity for the PPSV-23 vaccine. Although most users developed sufficient responses to both vaccines, administration of pneumococcal vaccine before initiation with tofacitinib may improve overall response and should be considered.

Clinical pearls: tofacitinib

- Patients should receive screening for tuberculosis before therapy initiation.
- Risk of herpes zoster may be higher in patients receiving tofacitinib, specifically Asian patients.
- Tofacitinib therapy may blunt the immune response to specific vaccines; therefore, patients should be assessed for appropriate immunizations before commencing therapy.

SPECIAL CONSIDERATIONS

Among the barriers to a successful arthritis treatment regimen is patient adherence to DMARD therapies. In this respect, illness beliefs and treatment beliefs may be more potent than socio-demographic factors and, therefore, amenable to clinician-based educational interventions.[94] One physician-related factor affecting adherence with therapy may include a focus on educational efforts that reinforce the belief that medication is necessary either for current or for future health.[95] Research efforts designed to assess whether or not the goal of achieving better control of inflammatory arthritis results in improved work participation is an area of academic need that would also support the goal of motivating enhanced patient adherence.[96]

Another area of future research with regard to the older rheumatology patient is the role of pharmacogenetics in disease susceptibility, severity, and response to treatment. Many of the DMARDs exhibit clinically significant differences in either efficacy or toxicity influenced by pharmacogenetic variants. For example, Moya and colleagues[97] recently showed that subjects with certain polymorphisms in genes responsible for methotrexate transport and metabolism exhibited a longer duration of methotrexate monotherapy and larger mean differences in the DAS score following 6 months of methotrexate monotherapy. Variants in folate transport and metabolism may influence the potential for methotrexate-related toxicities.[98] Pharmacogenetics may play a role in the development of HCQ-induced retinopathy, with 1 group finding an association between the development of retinopathy and mutations in the ABCR gene.[99] As previously mentioned, both SSZ and leflunomide also have pharmacogenetic-related considerations with regard to toxicity. As pharmacogenetics gains practical application, rheumatologists must partner with geriatricians to place this data into the appropriate context for optimal management of the older patient.

Finally, immunization strategies in older patients with rheumatologic conditions remain a conundrum for rheumatologists and primary care providers alike. Although current guidelines provide guidance on vaccine-related management for patients receiving selected DMARDs, biologic agents, and prednisone, these recommendations are often conditional in nature due to the lack of high-quality evidence in this area.[31,100] Additional studies are required to fully assess the safety and efficacy of vaccines, particularly live-virus vaccines, in older patients with rheumatological conditions receiving immunosuppressants, including traditional DMARDs and tofacitinib.

SUMMARY

In conclusion, a cohesive partnership between rheumatologists and geriatricians is crucial to the safe and effective management of older adults with rheumatologic conditions.

ACKNOWLEDGMENTS

The authors would like to thank Dr Adam Schiffenbauer for his critical reading and comments on this article.

REFERENCES

1. Summary health statistics: national health interview survey, 2014. 2014. Available at: http://ftp.cdc.gov/pub/Health_Statistics/NCHS/NHIS/SHS/2014_SHS_Table_A-4.pdf. Accessed January 15, 2016.
2. Helmick CG, Felson DT, Lawrence RC, et al. Estimates of the prevalence of arthritis and other rheumatic conditions in the United States. Part I. Arthritis Rheum 2008;58(1):15–25.
3. Budnitz DS, Pollock DA, Weidenbach KN, et al. National surveillance of emergency department visits for outpatient adverse drug events. JAMA 2006; 296(15):1858–66.
4. Baker DW, Gazmararian JA, Sudano J, et al. The association between age and health literacy among elderly persons. J Gerontol B Psychol Sci Soc Sci 2000; 55(6):S368–74.
5. Joplin S, van der Zwan R, Joshua F, et al. Medication adherence in patients with rheumatoid arthritis: the effect of patient education, health literacy, and musculoskeletal ultrasound. Biomed Res Int 2015;2015:150658.
6. Turnheim K. When drug therapy gets old: pharmacokinetics and pharmacodynamics in the elderly. Exp Gerontol 2003;38(8):843–53.
7. Ranganath VK, Furst DE. Disease-modifying antirheumatic drug use in the elderly rheumatoid arthritis patient. Rheum Dis Clin North Am 2007;33(1):197–217.
8. Shi S, Klotz U. Age-related changes in pharmacokinetics. Curr Drug Metab 2011;12(7):601–10.
9. Shah BM, Hajjar ER. Polypharmacy, adverse drug reactions, and geriatric syndromes. Clin Geriatr Med 2012;28(2):173–86.
10. Kievit W, van Hulst L, van Riel P, et al. Factors that influence rheumatologists' decisions to escalate care in rheumatoid arthritis: results from a choice-based conjoint analysis. Arthritis Care Res (Hoboken) 2010;62(6):842–7.
11. Juby A, Davis P. An evaluation of the impact of seniors on a rheumatology referral clinic: demographics and pharmacotherapy. Clin Rheumatol 2011; 30(11):1507–9.
12. Hovstadius B, Petersson G. Factors leading to excessive polypharmacy. Clin Geriatr Med 2012;28(2):159–72.
13. Hajjar ER, Cafiero AC, Hanlon JT. Polypharmacy in elderly patients. Am J Geriatr Pharmacother 2007;5(4):345–51.
14. Haider SI, Johnell K, Weitoft GR, et al. The influence of educational level on polypharmacy and inappropriate drug use: a register-based study of more than 600,000 older people. J Am Geriatr Soc 2009;57(1):62–9.
15. Treharne GJ, Douglas KM, Iwaszko J, et al. Polypharmacy among people with rheumatoid arthritis: the role of age, disease duration and comorbidity. Musculoskeletal Care 2007;5(4):175–90.

16. Viktil KK, Enstad M, Kutschera J, et al. Polypharmacy among patients admitted to hospital with rheumatic diseases. Pharm World Sci 2001;23(4):153–8.

17. Simonds SK. Health education as social policy. Health Educ Q 1974;2:1–10.

18. Wong PK, Christie L, Johnston J, et al. How well do patients understand written instructions?: health literacy assessment in rural and urban rheumatology outpatients. Medicine (Baltimore) 2014;93(25):e129.

19. Baker DW, Gazmararian JA, Williams MV, et al. Functional health literacy and the risk of hospital admission among Medicare managed care enrollees. Am J Public Health 2002;92(8):1278–83.

20. Buchbinder R, Hall S, Youd JM. Functional health literacy of patients with rheumatoid arthritis attending a community-based rheumatology practice. J Rheumatol 2006;33(5):879–86.

21. Caplan L, Wolfe F, Michaud K, et al. Strong association of health literacy with functional status among rheumatoid arthritis patients: a cross-sectional study. Arthritis Care Res (Hoboken) 2014;66(4):508–14.

22. Barton JL, Schmajuk G, Trupin L, et al. Poor knowledge of methotrexate associated with older age and limited English-language proficiency in a diverse rheumatoid arthritis cohort. Arthritis Res Ther 2013;15(5):R157.

23. Fraenkel L, Rabidou N, Dhar R. Are rheumatologists' treatment decisions influenced by patients' age? Rheumatology (Oxford) 2006;45(12):1555–7.

24. Radovits BJ, Fransen J, Eijsbouts A, et al. Missed opportunities in the treatment of elderly patients with rheumatoid arthritis. Rheumatology (Oxford) 2009;48(8):906–10.

25. Koller MD, Aletaha D, Funovits J, et al. Response of elderly patients with rheumatoid arthritis to methotrexate or TNF inhibitors compared with younger patients. Rheumatology (Oxford) 2009;48(12):1575–80.

26. Gubner R, August S, Ginsberg V. Therapeutic suppression of tissue reactivity. II. Effect of aminopterin in rheumatoid arthritis and psoriasis. Am J Med Sci 1951;221(2):176–82.

27. Gubner R. Therapeutic suppression of tissue reactivity I. Comparison of the effects of cortisone and aminopterin. Am J Med Sci 1951;221(2):169–75.

28. Weinblatt ME, Kaplan H, Germain BF, et al. Methotrexate in rheumatoid arthritis: effects on disease activity in a multicenter prospective study. J Rheumatol 1991;18(3):334–8.

29. Wolfe F, Cathey MA. The effect of age on methotrexate efficacy and toxicity. J Rheumatol 1991;18(7):973–7.

30. The effect of age and renal function on the efficacy and toxicity of methotrexate in rheumatoid arthritis. Rheumatoid Arthritis Clinical Trial Archive Group. J Rheumatol 1995;22(2):218–23.

31. Singh JA, Saag KG, Bridges SL Jr, et al. 2015 American college of rheumatology guideline for the treatment of rheumatoid arthritis. Arthritis Rheumatol 2016;68(1):1–26.

32. Cronstein BN. The mechanism of action of methotrexate. Rheum Dis Clin North Am 1997;23(4):739–55.

33. Davila L, Ranganathan P. Pharmacogenetics: implications for therapy in rheumatic diseases. Nat Rev Rheumatol 2011;7(9):537–50.

34. Visser K, van der Heijde D. Optimal dosage and route of administration of methotrexate in rheumatoid arthritis: a systematic review of the literature. Ann Rheum Dis 2009;68(7):1094–9.

35. Schiff MH, Jaffe JS, Freundlich B. Head-to-head, randomised, crossover study of oral versus subcutaneous methotrexate in patients with rheumatoid

arthritis: drug-exposure limitations of oral methotrexate at doses >/=15 mg may be overcome with subcutaneous administration. Ann Rheum Dis 2014; 73(8):1549–51.

36. Bressolle F, Bologna C, Kinowski JM, et al. Effects of moderate renal insufficiency on pharmacokinetics of methotrexate in rheumatoid arthritis patients. Ann Rheum Dis 1998;57(2):110–3.

37. Alarcon GS, Tracy IC, Blackburn WD Jr. Methotrexate in rheumatoid arthritis. Toxic effects as the major factor in limiting long-term treatment. Arthritis Rheum 1989;32(6):671–6.

38. Lim AY, Gaffney K, Scott DG. Methotrexate-induced pancytopenia: serious and under-reported? Our experience of 25 cases in 5 years. Rheumatology (Oxford) 2005;44(8):1051–5.

39. Felson DT, Anderson JJ, Meenan RF. Use of short-term efficacy/toxicity tradeoffs to select second-line drugs in rheumatoid arthritis. A metaanalysis of published clinical trials. Arthritis Rheum 1992;35(10):1117–25.

40. Shea B, Swinden MV, Tanjong Ghogomu E, et al. Folic acid and folinic acid for reducing side effects in patients receiving methotrexate for rheumatoid arthritis. Cochrane Database Syst Rev 2013;(5):CD000951.

41. Dhir V, Sandhu A, Kaur J, et al. Comparison of two different folic acid doses with methotrexate–a randomized controlled trial (FOLVARI Study). Arthritis Res Ther 2015;17:156.

42. Diaz-Borjon A. Guidelines for the use of conventional and newer disease-modifying antirheumatic drugs in elderly patients with rheumatoid arthritis. Drugs Aging 2009;26(4):273–93.

43. Bourre-Tessier J, Haraoui B. Methotrexate drug interactions in the treatment of rheumatoid arthritis: a systematic review. J Rheumatol 2010;37(7):1416–21.

44. Wang GY, Zhang SL, Wang XR, et al. Remission of rheumatoid arthritis and potential determinants: a national multi-center cross-sectional survey. Clin Rheumatol 2015;34(2):221–30.

45. Moreland LW, O'Dell JR, Paulus HE, et al. A randomized comparative effectiveness study of oral triple therapy versus etanercept plus methotrexate in early aggressive rheumatoid arthritis: the treatment of Early Aggressive Rheumatoid Arthritis Trial. Arthritis Rheum 2012;64(9):2824–35.

46. A randomized study of the effect of withdrawing hydroxychloroquine sulfate in systemic lupus erythematosus. The Canadian Hydroxychloroquine Study Group. N Engl J Med 1991;324(3):150–4.

47. Alarcon GS, McGwin G, Bertoli AM, et al. Effect of hydroxychloroquine on the survival of patients with systemic lupus erythematosus: data from LUMINA, a multiethnic US cohort (LUMINA L). Ann Rheum Dis 2007;66(9):1168–72.

48. Cohen PR. Hydroxychloroquine-associated hyperpigmentation mimicking elder abuse. Dermatol Ther (heidelb) 2013;3(2):203–10.

49. True DG, Bryant LR, Harris MD, et al. Clinical images: hydroxychloroquine-associated mucocutaneous hyperpigmentation. Arthritis Rheum 2002;46(6):1698.

50. Wolfe F, Marmor MF. Rates and predictors of hydroxychloroquine retinal toxicity in patients with rheumatoid arthritis and systemic lupus erythematosus. Arthritis Care Res (Hoboken) 2010;62(6):775–84.

51. Melles RB, Marmor MF. The risk of toxic retinopathy in patients on long-term hydroxychloroquine therapy. JAMA Ophthalmol 2014;132(12):1453–60.

52. Marmor MF, Kellner U, Lai TY, et al, American Academy of Ophthalmology. Revised recommendations on screening for chloroquine and hydroxychloroquine retinopathy. Ophthalmology 2011;118(2):415–22.

53. Jallouli M, Galicier L, Zahr N, et al. Determinants of hydroxychloroquine blood concentration variations in systemic lupus erythematosus. Arthritis Rheumatol 2015;67(8):2176–84.
54. Lee JY, Luc S, Greenblatt DJ, et al. Factors associated with blood hydroxychloroquine level in lupus patients: renal function could be important. Lupus 2013; 22(5):541–2.
55. Biehl A, Ghaderi - Yeganeh M, Manna Z, et al. Hydroxychloroquine level variants and predictors in a connective tissue disease population [abstract]. Arthritis Rheumatol 2015;67(Suppl 10):2186.
56. Costedoat-Chalumeau N, Amoura Z, Hulot JS, et al. Very low blood hydroxy-chloroquine concentration as an objective marker of poor adherence to treatment of systemic lupus erythematosus. Ann Rheum Dis 2007;66(6):821–4.
57. van der Heijde D, Sieper J, Elewaut D, et al. Referral patterns, diagnosis, and disease management of patients with axial spondyloarthritis: results of an international survey. J Clin Rheumatol 2014;20(8):411–7.
58. Eriksson JK, Karlsson JA, Bratt J, et al. Cost-effectiveness of infliximab versus conventional combination treatment in methotrexate-refractory early rheumatoid arthritis: 2-year results of the register-enriched randomised controlled SWEFOT trial. Ann Rheum Dis 2015;74(6):1094–101.
59. van der Heijde D, Zack D, Wajdula J, et al. Rates of serious infections, opportunistic infections, inflammatory bowel disease, and malignancies in subjects receiving etanercept vs. controls from clinical trials in ankylosing spondylitis: a pooled analysis. Scand J Rheumatol 2014;43(1):49–53.
60. Kim SC, Yelin E, Tonner C, et al. Changes in use of disease-modifying antirheumatic drugs for rheumatoid arthritis in the United States during 1983-2009. Arthritis Care Res (Hoboken) 2013;65(9):1529–33.
61. Greenberg JD, Palmer JB, Li Y, et al. Healthcare resource use and direct costs in patients with ankylosing spondylitis and psoriatic arthritis in a large US cohort. J Rheumatol 2016;43(1):88–96.
62. Tarnowski M, Paradowska-Gorycka A, Dabrowska-Zamojcin E, et al. The effect of gene polymorphisms on patient responses to rheumatoid arthritis therapy. Expert Opin Drug Metab Toxicol 2016;12(1):41–55.
63. Cummins L, Katikireddi VS, Shankaranarayana S, et al. Safety and retention of combination triple disease-modifying anti-rheumatic drugs in new-onset rheumatoid arthritis. Intern Med J 2015;45(12):1266–73.
64. Mechanick JI. Coombs' positive hemolytic anemia following sulfasalazine therapy in ulcerative colitis: case reports, review, and discussion of pathogenesis. Mt Sinai J Med 1985;52(8):667–70.
65. Okubo S, Nakatani K, Nishiya K. Gastrointestinal symptoms associated with enteric-coated sulfasalazine (Azulfidine EN tablets). Mod Rheumatol 2002; 12(3):226–9.
66. Weaver A, Chatwell R, Churchill M, et al. Improved gastrointestinal tolerance and patient preference of enteric-coated sulfasalazine versus uncoated sulfasalazine tablets in patients with rheumatoid arthritis. J Clin Rheumatol 1999;5(4): 193–200.
67. Raithatha N, Mehrtens S, Mouyis M, et al. Rash and fever after sulfasalazine use. BMJ 2014;349:g5655.
68. Mun JI, Shin SJ, Yu BH, et al. A case of hemophagocytic syndrome in a patient with fulminant ulcerative colitis superinfected by cytomegalovirus. Korean J Intern Med 2013;28(3):352–5.

69. DeMichele J, Rezaizadeh H, Goldstein JI. Sulfasalazine crystalluria-induced anuric renal failure. Clin Gastroenterol Hepatol 2012;10(2):A32.

70. Sands K, Jansen R, Zaslau S, et al. Review article: the safety of therapeutic drugs in male inflammatory bowel disease patients wishing to conceive. Aliment Pharmacol Ther 2015;41(9):821–34.

71. Fragoso YD, Brooks JB. Leflunomide and teriflunomide: altering the metabolism of pyrimidines for the treatment of autoimmune diseases. Expert Rev Clin Pharmacol 2015;8(3):315–20.

72. Alivernini S, Mazzotta D, Zoli A, et al. Leflunomide treatment in elderly patients with rheumatoid or psoriatic arthritis: retrospective analysis of safety and adherence to treatment. Drugs Aging 2009;26(5):395–402.

73. Baker JF, Sauer BC, Cannon GW, et al. Changes in Body Mass Related to the Initiation of Disease-Modifying Therapies in Rheumatoid Arthritis. Arthritis Rheumatol 2016;68(8):1818–27.

74. Hopkins AM, Wiese MD, Proudman SM, et al. Genetic polymorphism of CYP1A2 but not total or free teriflunomide concentrations is associated with leflunomide cessation in rheumatoid arthritis. Br J Clin Pharmacol 2016;81(1):113–23.

75. Wiese MD, Schnabl M, O'Doherty C, et al. Polymorphisms in cytochrome P450 2C19 enzyme and cessation of leflunomide in patients with rheumatoid arthritis. Arthritis Res Ther 2012;14(4):R163.

76. Rozman B. Clinical pharmacokinetics of leflunomide. Clin Pharmacokinet 2002; 41(6):421–30.

77. Wong SP, Chu CM, Kan CH, et al. Successful treatment of leflunomide-induced acute pneumonitis with cholestyramine wash-out therapy. J Clin Rheumatol 2009;15(8):389–92.

78. Laub M, Fraser R, Kurche J, et al. Use of a cholestyramine washout in a patient with septic shock on leflunomide therapy: a case report and review of the literature. J Intensive Care Med 2016;31(6):412–4.

79. Hajdyla-Banas I, Banas T, Rydz-Stryszowska I, et al. Pregnancy course and neonatal outcome after exposure to leflunomide–2 cases report and review of literature. Przegl Lek 2009;66(12):1069–71.

80. O'Shea JJ, Schwartz DM, Villarino AV, et al. The JAK-STAT pathway: impact on human disease and therapeutic intervention. Annu Rev Med 2015;66:311–28.

81. Tanaka Y, Suzuki M, Nakamura H, et al, Tofacitinib Study I. Phase II study of tofacitinib (CP-690,550) combined with methotrexate in patients with rheumatoid arthritis and an inadequate response to methotrexate. Arthritis Care Res (Hoboken) 2011;63(8):1150–8.

82. Fleischmann R, Cutolo M, Genovese MC, et al. Phase IIb dose-ranging study of the oral JAK inhibitor tofacitinib (CP-690,550) or adalimumab monotherapy versus placebo in patients with active rheumatoid arthritis with an inadequate response to disease-modifying antirheumatic drugs. Arthritis Rheum 2012; 64(3):617–29.

83. Fleischmann R, Kremer J, Cush J, et al. Placebo-controlled trial of tofacitinib monotherapy in rheumatoid arthritis. N Engl J Med 2012;367(6):495–507.

84. Kremer JM, Cohen S, Wilkinson BE, et al. A phase IIb dose-ranging study of the oral JAK inhibitor tofacitinib (CP-690,550) versus placebo in combination with background methotrexate in patients with active rheumatoid arthritis and an inadequate response to methotrexate alone. Arthritis Rheum 2012;64(4): 970–81.

85. Vincenti F, Tedesco Silva H, Busque S, et al. Randomized phase 2b trial of tofacitinib (CP-690,550) in de novo kidney transplant patients: efficacy, renal function and safety at 1 year. Am J Transplant 2012;12(9):2446–56.
86. Sandborn WJ, Ghosh S, Panes J, et al. Tofacitinib, an oral Janus kinase inhibitor, in active ulcerative colitis. N Engl J Med 2012;367(7):616–24.
87. Craiglow BG, King BA. Killing two birds with one stone: oral tofacitinib reverses alopecia universalis in a patient with plaque psoriasis. J Invest Dermatol 2014; 134(12):2988–90.
88. Xeljanz (R) [package insert]. New York: Pfizer Labs; 2016.
89. Wollenhaupt J, Silverfield J, Lee EB, et al. Safety and efficacy of tofacitinib, an oral janus kinase inhibitor, for the treatment of rheumatoid arthritis in open-label, longterm extension studies. J Rheumatol 2014;41(5):837–52.
90. Strand V, Ahadieh S, French J, et al. Systematic review and meta-analysis of serious infections with tofacitinib and biologic disease-modifying antirheumatic drug treatment in rheumatoid arthritis clinical trials. Arthritis Res Ther 2015; 17(1):362.
91. Winthrop KL, Yamanaka H, Valdez H, et al. Herpes zoster and tofacitinib therapy in patients with rheumatoid arthritis. Arthritis Rheumatol 2014;66(10):2675–84.
92. Zhang J, Delzell E, Xie F, et al. The use, safety, and effectiveness of herpes zoster vaccination in individuals with inflammatory and autoimmune diseases: a longitudinal observational study. Arthritis Res Ther 2011;13(5):R174.
93. Winthrop KL, Silverfield J, Racewicz A, et al. The effect of tofacitinib on pneumococcal and influenza vaccine responses in rheumatoid arthritis. Ann Rheum Dis 2015;75(4):687–95.
94. Kumar K, Raza K, Nightingale P, et al. Determinants of adherence to disease modifying anti-rheumatic drugs in White British and South Asian patients with rheumatoid arthritis: a cross sectional study. BMC Musculoskelet Disord 2015; 16:396.
95. Foot H, La Caze A, Gujral G, et al. The necessity-concerns framework predicts adherence to medication in multiple illness conditions: a meta-analysis. Patient Educ Couns 2015;99(5):706–17.
96. Palmer KT, Goodson N. Ageing, musculoskeletal health and work. Best Pract Res Clin Rheumatol 2015;29(3):391–404.
97. Moya P, Salazar J, Arranz MJ, et al. Methotrexate pharmacokinetic genetic variants are associated with outcome in rheumatoid arthritis patients. Pharmacogenomics 2016;17(1):25–9.
98. Berkun Y, Levartovsky D, Rubinow A, et al. Methotrexate related adverse effects in patients with rheumatoid arthritis are associated with the A1298C polymorphism of the MTHFR gene. Ann Rheum Dis 2004;63(10):1227–31.
99. Shroyer NF, Lewis RA, Lupski JR. Analysis of the ABCR (ABCA4) gene in 4-aminoquinoline retinopathy: is retinal toxicity by chloroquine and hydroxychloroquine related to Stargardt disease? Am J Ophthalmol 2001;131(6):761–6.
100. Hales CM, Harpaz R, Ortega-Sanchez I, et al. Update on recommendations for use of herpes zoster vaccine. MMWR Morb Mortal Wkly Rep 2014;63(33): 729–31.

Pathogenesis and Management of Sarcopenia

 CrossMark

Robinder J.S. Dhillon, MD, MBA, Sarfaraz Hasni, MD*

KEYWORDS

- Sarcopenia • Muscle strength • Muscle atrophy • Frailty • Aging • Senescence
- Fall risk • Skeletal muscle mass loss

KEY POINTS

- Sarcopenia is a prevalent but under-recognized problem in the elderly population, causing limitation of activities of daily living and increasing the risk of fall and mortality.
- To date, a common clinical definition and diagnostic criteria for sarcopenia are lacking. The most commonly used screening tool developed by the European Working Group on Sarcopenia in Older People has several limitations but is endorsed by many professional medical societies.
- The goal of this article is to promote awareness among physicians of early recognition of sarcopenia and its management in the geriatric patient population.

INTRODUCTION

The term Sarcopenia (Greek, *sarx* for:"flesh" and *penia* for "loss") refers to the phenomenon of reduction of both muscular mass and function with aging.[1] Muscle strength is a critical component of walking, and its decrease in the elderly contributes to a high prevalence of falls. Sarcopenia is significantly associated with self-reported physical disability in both men and women, independent of ethnicity, age, morbidity, obesity, income, or health behaviors.[2] Reduced muscle strength with aging leads to loss of functional capacity and is a major cause of disability, mortality, and other adverse health outcomes.[3] As the number and proportion of older persons in the population continue to rise, sarcopenia-related morbidity will become an increasing area of health care resource utilization.

Initial descriptions of sarcopenia focused on loss of muscle mass and did not consider inclusion of muscle strength or physical impairment as part of the disease

Disclosure Statement: This research was supported by the Intramural Research Program of the National Institute of Arthritis and Musculoskeletal and Skin Diseases of the National Institutes of Health.
National Institute of Arthritis and Musculoskeletal and Skin Diseases, National Institutes of Health, 9000 Rockville Pike, Building 10, Room Number 3-2340, Bethesda, MD 20892, USA
* Corresponding author.
E-mail address: hasnisa@mail.nih.gov

process.[3] The 2010 European Working Group on Sarcopenia in Older People (EWG-SOP) recognized that muscle strength and muscle mass are significant components of sarcopenia. The group defined sarcopenia as a syndrome characterized by progressive and generalized loss of skeletal muscle mass and strength with risk of adverse outcomes such as physical disability, poor quality of life, and death.[4–6] Early recognition and intervention can mitigate some of these deleterious outcomes.

EPIDEMIOLOGY

There is a significant variability in the reported prevalence of sarcopenia. A recent study of community-dwelling older adults (average age of 67 years) in the United Kingdom found the sarcopenia prevalence to be 4.6% in men and 7.9% in women using the EWGSOP criteria.[7] A study from the United States, conducted among older adults with an average age of 70.1 years, reported the prevalence of sarcopenia to be as high as 36.5%.[8] In a Japanese population of community-dwelling elderly adults, the prevalence of sarcopenia ranged from 2.5% to 28.0% in men and 2.3% to 11.7% in women (using dual-energy X-ray absorptiometry [DEXA] for measuring lean body mass), and 7.1% to 98.0% in men and 19.8% to 88.0% in women (measured by bioelectrical impedance analysis).[9] In a large cohort of 2867 community-dwelling older adults (age >65 years) in Taiwan, the prevalence of sarcopenia varied from 3.9% to 7.3% with prevalence reaching 13.6% among men aged 75 years and older.[10] Much of the difference in these estimates may be due to the lack of uniform criteria to diagnose sarcopenia.

RISK FACTORS

Sarcopenia is considered by most to be an inevitable part of aging. However, the degree of sarcopenia is highly variable and is dependent upon the presence of certain risk factors.

Lifestyle Lacking Exercise

Lack of exercise is believed to be the foremost risk factor for sarcopenia.[11] A gradual decline in muscle fiber numbers begins around 50 years of age.[12] The decline in muscle fiber and strength is more pronounced in patients with sedentary lifestyle as compared to patients who are physically more active. Even professional athletes such as marathon runners and weight lifters show a gradual, albeit more slower, decline in their speed and strength with aging.[12]

Hormone and Cytokine Imbalance

Age-related decreases in hormone concentrations, including growth hormone, testosterone, thyroid hormone, and insulin-like growth factor, lead to loss of muscle mass and strength. Extreme muscle loss often results from a combination of diminishing hormonal anabolic signals and promotion of catabolic signals mediated through proinflammatory cytokines such as tumor necrosis factor alpha (TNF-α) and interleukin-6 (IL-6).[13] Elevated levels of both TNF-α and IL-6 have been shown to be present in skeletal muscles of older individuals.

Protein Synthesis and Regeneration

A decrease in the body's ability to synthesize protein, coupled with inadequate intake of calories and/or protein to sustain muscle mass, is common in sarcopenia. Oxidized proteins increase in skeletal muscle with aging and lead to a buildup of lipofuscin and cross-linked proteins that are inadequately removed via the proteolysis system. This leads to an accumulation of noncontractile dysfunctional protein in skeletal muscles, and is part of the reason muscle strength decreases severely in sarcopenia.[14]

Motor Unit Remodelling

Age-related reduction in motor nerve cells responsible for sending signals from the brain to the muscles to initiate movement also occurs. Satellite cells are small mono-nuclear cells that abut muscle fibers and are normally activated upon injury or exercise. In response to these signals, satellite cells differentiate and fuse into the muscle fiber, helping to maintain muscle function. One current hypothesis is that sarcopenia is caused, in part, by a failure in satellite cell activation.[13]

Evolutionary Basis

Evolutionary theories implicate the failure of the body to maintain muscle mass and function with aging on genes that govern these traits. This hypothesis suggests that genes suited for high levels of obligatory muscular effort required for survival in the Late Paleolithic epoch are ill-matched to a modern lifestyle characterized by high levels of lifelong sedentary behavior.[15]

Early Developmental Influences

Epidemiologic research into the developmental origins of health and disease has shown that early environmental influences on growth and development may have long-term consequences for human health. Low birth weight, a marker of a poor early environment, is associated with reduced muscle mass and strength in adult life.[16,17] One study has shown that lower birth weight is associated with a significant decrease in muscle fiber score, suggesting that developmental influences on muscle morphology may explain the association between low birth weight and sarcopenia.[18]

DIAGNOSING SARCOPENIA

The evaluation of sarcopenia requires objective measurements of muscle strength and muscle mass. Several methods of evaluating sarcopenia currently used include walking speed, calf circumference (CC), bioimpedance analysis (BIA), handgrip strength, DEXA, and imaging methods (computerized tomography and magnetic resonance imaging). None of these measures are very sensitive or specific for evaluating sarcopenia.[19,20]

In 1998, Baumgartner and colleagues[2] proposed using lean body mass, as determined by DEXA, compared with a normal reference population as a standard measure for sarcopenia. His working definition used a cut-off point of 2 standard deviations below the mean of lean mass for gender-specific healthy young adults.

This methodology showed promise, being both practical and predictive for negative outcomes.[2] Moreover, given its similarity to the 1996 World Health Organization (WHO) DEXA methodology for diagnosing osteoporosis, the same scan used in osteoporosis screening may be used to estimate the degree of sarcopenia with no added cost or radiation exposure to the patient. However, this method has several limitations, such as the ability of DEXA to distinguish water retention or fat infiltration within muscle or the muscle mass in relation to total body mass. Subsequently, other researchers have proposed various methods to account for these limitations; but to date there is no universally accepted method to diagnose sarcopenia.

This initial definition of sarcopenia was further modified by the European Society on Clinician Nutrition and Metabolism (ESPEN) special interest groups (SIGs) on geriatric nutrition and on cachexia–anorexia in chronic wasting diseases.[21] Sarcopenia was defined as the following (consensus statement)

1. A low muscle mass, greater than 2 standard deviations below that mean measured in young adults (aged 18–39 years in the third NHANES [National Health and Nutrition Examination Survey] population) of the same sex and ethnic background
2. Low gait speed (eg, a walking speed below 0.8 m/s in the 4-minute walking test).

More recently, EWGSOP proposed the following diagnostic criteria for sarcopenia[6]:

1. Low muscle mass (LMM), assessed by skeletal muscle mass index of no more than 8.90 kg/m^2 (men) and 6.37 kg/m^2 (women);
2. Low muscle strength (LMS) assessed by handgrip strength less than 30 kg (men) and 20 kg (women)
3. Low physical performance (LPP) assessed by gait speed of no more than ≤0.8 m/s

A detailed description of methods to determine LMM, LMS, and LPP are well described in the literature.[22] The diagnosis of sarcopenia required the presence of LMM plus LMS or LPP.

In addition, the EWGSOP suggested staging of sarcopenia into 3 different categories based upon the presence of LMM and the presence or absence of functional impairment[6] (**Table 1**).

These progressive stages of sarcopenia have a dose–response relationship with functional limitations.

SARCOPENIA HISTOPATHOLOGY

Early sarcopenia is characterized by a decrease in the size of muscle. Over time, a reduction in muscle tissue quality also occurs. This is characterized by replacement of muscle fibers with fat, an increase in fibrosis, changes in muscle metabolism, oxidative stress, and degeneration of the neuromuscular junction. This ultimately leads to progressive loss of muscle function and to frailty.[13]

Studies looking at the histologic changes in muscle fibers reveal that sarcopenia predominantly effects the type II (fast-twitch) muscle fibers, whereas type I (slow-twitch) fibers are much less affected.[23] The size of type II fibers can be reduced by up to 50% in sarcopenia. However, such reductions are only moderate when compared with overall reductions in muscle mass. This raises the possibility that sarcopenia represents both a reduction in muscle fiber number as well as reduced fiber size. Histologic studies comparing muscle cross-sections of elderly with those of younger individuals reveal at least 50% fewer type I and type II fibers by the ninth decade.[24] Results from anatomic and electrophysiological studies demonstrate loss of anterior horn cells and ventral root fibers with aging.[25,26] The mechanism of these

Table 1 Staging of sarcopenia			
Stage	Muscle Mass	Muscle Strength	Performance
Presarcopenia	Low	Normal	Normal
Sarcopenia	Low	Low	Normal or low
Severe sarcopenia	Low	Low	Low

From Cruz-Jentoft AJ, Baeyens JP, Bauer JM, et al. Sarcopenia: European consensus on definition and diagnosis: report of the European Working Group on Sarcopenia in Older People. Age Aging 2010;39(4):414; with permission.

histologic changes may suggest that a chronic neuropathic process contributes to a loss of motor neurons that leads to reduced muscle mass. Other factors such as lifestyle, hormones, inflammatory cytokines, and genetic factors also influence these histologic changes.

MANAGEMENT

Early recognition and intervention are key to improved outcomes in patients with sarcopenia. Screening patients for impairment in their physical function and activities of daily living (ADLs) should be a routine part of health care visits for the elderly. Patients with impaired ADLs should undergo more specific testing for sarcopenia. Assessment of patients' environments for fall hazards and implementation of precautionary safety measures should be part of the treatment strategy.

Nonpharmacologic Treatment

Physical inactivity is linked to loss of muscle strength and mass. Therefore an exercise regimen is considered a cornerstone in the treatment of sarcopenia. Short-term resistance exercise has been demonstrated to increase ability and capacity of skeletal muscle to synthesize proteins.[27] Both resistance training (RT) and strength training (ST) of muscles have been shown to be somewhat successful interventions in the prevention and treatment of sarcopenia. RT has been reported to positively influence the neuromuscular system and increase hormone concentrations and the rate of protein synthesis.[28] A recent meta-analysis revealed some benefit of using a combined approach of dietary supplements and exercise, but the findings were inconsistent among various populations.[29]

Pharmacological Therapies

Currently, there are no agents for the treatment of sarcopenia that have been approved by the US Food and Drug Administration. DeHydroEpiAndrosterone (DHEA) and human growth hormone have little to no effect. Growth hormone increases muscle protein synthesis and increases muscle mass but does not lead to gains in strength and function. This, and the similar lack of efficacy of its effector, insulin-like growth factor 1 (IGF-1), may be due to local resistance to IGF-1 in aging muscle that results from inflammation and other age-related changes.[30]

Testosterone an other anabolic steroids have also been investigated. These agents have a modest positive effect on muscle strength and mass but are of limited use due to adverse effects, such as increased risk of prostate cancer in men, virilization in women, and an overall increased risk of cardiovascular events.[30,31]

New therapies for sarcopenia are in clinical development. Selective androgen receptor modulators (SARMs) are of particular interest because of their tissue selectivity. It is hoped that androgenic signaling with these agents can achieve gains in skeletal muscle mass and strength without dose-limiting adverse events.[32] Other compounds under investigation as treatments for sarcopenia include myostatin, vitamin D, angiotensin-converting enzyme inhibitors, eicosapentaenoic acid,[30,31] thalidomide, OHR/AVR118, celecoxib, VT-122, omega-3 supplements, and anabolic agents such as ghrelin and its analogues, MT-102, BYM338, and ruxolotinib.[33] MT-102, the first-in-class anabolic catabolic-transforming agent (ACTA), has recently been tested in a phase II clinical study for treating cachexia in late-stage cancer patients. The study data show significant increases in body weight in patients treated with 10 mg of MT-102 twice daily over the study period of 16 weeks, compared with a significant decrease in body weight in patients receiving placebo treatment.[34] In aged animal models, MT-102 has been shown to reverse sarcopenia.[35] Further studies of MT-102 as a treatment of sarcopenia are currently underway. Another clinical trial using intravenous BYM338 (bimagrumab) in patients with sarcopenia is currently enrolling subjects.[36]

Herbal Supplements and Nutrition

There is a great deal of interest in using herbal supplements to promote muscular mass and health in patients with sarcopenia. A recent review reported a large number of herbal compounds with effects on skeletal muscles.[37] Some of the herbal compounds showed modest effects on skeletal muscle in human studies. These include curcumin from *Curcuma longa*, alkaloids and steroidal lactones from *Withania somnifera*, catechins from *Camellia sinensis*, proanthocyanidin of grape seeds, and gingerols and shogaols from *Zingiber officinale*.[37] The data supporting use of these supplements in people are limited as pertains to efficacy, as well as potential drug interactions and adverse effects. Hence, support for the use of herbal supplements for treatment and prevention of sarcopenia is limited until further research proves their safety and efficacy in people.

Malnutrition also contributes to the development of sarcopenia. Nutritional screening and implementation of nutrition care plans similar to the approach to cachexia should be part of a multidisciplinary approach to manage sarcopenia.[38] A validated tool for nutritional needs assessment developed by The British Association for Parenteral and Enteral Nutrition is available online at www.bapen.org.uk.[39] Finally, high protein intake above the recommended daily allowance (in the range of 1.2–1.6 g/kg/d) has been suggested to prevent age-related sarcopenia.[40]

SECONDARY SARCOPENIA

Sarcopenia is often related to other underlying medical conditions. The pathogenic mechanisms that cause muscle wasting in secondary sarcopenia can provide useful insights into age-related sarcopenia. The management of secondary sarcopenia should focus on treating the underlying primary condition, with the same strategies to improve skeletal muscle strength and mass outlined previously.

Cachexia

Cachexia is characterized by severe muscle wasting usually accompanying severe systemic diseases such as cancer, cardiomyopathy, and end-stage renal disease.[41] Cachexia has recently been defined as a complex metabolic syndrome associated with underlying illness and characterized by loss of muscle with or without loss of fat mass.[42] Cachexia is frequently associated with inflammation, insulin resistance, anorexia, and increased breakdown of muscle proteins.[43,44] Thus, most cachectic individuals are also sarcopenic, but most sarcopenic individuals are not considered cachectic. Sarcopenia is among the elements of the proposed definition for cachexia.[42] Recently, a consensus definition to differentiate between cachexia and other conditions associated with sarcopenia was developed by the special interest group on cachexia–anorexia in chronic wasting diseases of the European Society for Clinical Nutrition and Metabolism (ESPEN-SIG).[21]

Frailty

Frailty is a geriatric syndrome resulting from age-related cumulative declines across multiple physiologic systems, with impaired homeostatic reserve and a reduced capacity of the organism to withstand stress. The syndrome encompasses increased vulnerability to adverse health outcomes such as falls, hospitalization, institutionaliza-tion, and mortality.[45] Frailty is based upon readily identifiable physical impairments, with the presence of 3 or more of the following characteristics: unintended weight loss, exhaustion, weakness, slow gait speed, and low physical activity.[45,46] There ex-ists significant overlap between frailty and sarcopenia; most frail older people have sarcopenia, which suggests a common pathogenic mechanism. The general concept of frailty, however, goes beyond physical factors to encompass psychological and so-cial dimensions as well. This may include cognitive decline, lack of social support, and the impact of the local environment.[46]

Sarcopenic Obesity

Sarcopenic obesity (SO) is a medical condition in which low lean body mass seen in sarcopenia is coupled with high fat mass. It is associated with impaired functional ca-pacity, disability, metabolic complications, and mortality.[47] The reported prevalence of SO is between 2% to 21.7%. The likely explanation for wide variability in reported prevalence is due to factors such as lack of awareness of SO among health care pro-viders and differences in genetics, nutrition, and lifestyle.[48] In conditions such as ma-lignancy and rheumatoid arthritis, lean body mass may be lost while fat mass is preserved or increased.[47] Low muscle mass along with high fat mass may also be characteristic of the aging process. However, the presence of SO in older individuals poses a diagnostic challenge, because the age-related reduction of muscle mass and strength may be independent of body mass index.

It has long been thought that the age-related loss of weight, along with a loss of muscle mass, was largely responsible for muscle weakness in older people.[49] How-ever, studies in patients with SO reveal that changes in muscle composition are also important. Marbling, or fat infiltration into muscle, lowers muscle quality and work performance.[50] Studies to understand the pathogenesis of SO observed certain patterns of age-related changes in body muscle and fat composition. In aging men, the percentage of fat mass increases initially and later levels off or decreases.[50] There is a redistribution of fat that occurs with aging as well, characterized by an increase in intramuscular and visceral fat, with a reduction in subcutaneous fat.[51,52] Such changes may play a role in the development of SO.

SUMMARY AND FUTURE DIRECTION

Sarcopenia is a growing global health concern. Sarcopenia has been reported to affect 5% to 13% of persons aged 60 to 70 years and up to 50% of people over 80 years of age.[53] In 2000, the number of people at least 60 years old around the world was estimated to be 600 million. This population is expected to rise to 1.2 billion by 2025 and 2 billion by 2050.[54] Even with a conservative estimate of prevalence, sarco-penia affects more than 50 million people today and will affect more than 200 million people in the next 40 years.

The diagnosis of sarcopenia can be difficult to affirm. The comprehensive measure-ments used in research are not always practical in health care settings and do not typi-cally influence care planning. Exercise remains the intervention of choice for managing sarcopenia, but implementing an exercise program may be challenging for many rea-sons. The role of nutrition in preventing and treating sarcopenia is less clear. Although there is vigorous debate about what level of protein intake is optimal, ensuring adequate protein intake and replacing deficient nutrients and vitamins are recommended.[55,56]

Future research should focus on exploring the biological pathways that lead to sar-copenia, along with the search for improved diagnostic biomarkers. Increased awareness among patients and health care providers, early screening, and a multidisciplinary approach to treatment are the best current practices to minimize the overall adverse impact of sarcopenia.[57]

REFERENCES

1. Rosenberg IH. Sarcopenia: origins and clinical relevance. J Nutr 1997;127(5 Suppl):990S–1S.
2. Baumgartner RN, Koehler KM, Gallagher D, et al. Epidemiology of sarcopenia among the elderly in New Mexico. Am J Epidemiol 1998;147(8):755–63.
3. Roubenoff R. Origins and clinical relevance of sarcopenia. Can J Appl Physiol 2001;26(1):78–89.
4. Goodpaster BH, Park SW, Harris TB, et al. The loss of skeletal muscle strength, mass, and quality in older adults: the health, aging and body composition study. J Gerontol A Biol Sci Med Sci 2006;61(10):1059–64.
5. Delmonico MJ, Harris TB, Lee JS, et al. Alternative definitions of sarcopenia, lower extremity performance, and functional impairment with aging in older men and women. J Am Geriatr Soc 2007;55(5):769–74.
6. Cruz-Jentoft AJ, Baeyens JP, Bauer JM, et al. Sarcopenia: European consensus on definition and diagnosis: report of the European working group on Sarcopenia in older people. Age Ageing 2010;39(4):412–23.
7. Patel HP, Syddall HE, Jameson K, et al. Prevalence of sarcopenia in community-dwelling older people in the UK using the European working group on sarcopenia in older people (EWGSOP) definition: findings from the Hertfordshire Cohort Study (HCS). Age Ageing 2013;42(3):378–84.
8. Brown JC, Harhay MO, Harhay MN. Sarcopenia and mortality among a population-based sample of community-dwelling older adults. J Cachexia Sarcopenia Muscle 2016;7(3):290–8.
9. Kim H, Hirano H, Edahiro A, et al. Sarcopenia: prevalence and associated factors based on different suggested definitions in community-dwelling older adults. Geriatr Gerontol Int 2016;16(Suppl 1):110–22.
10. Wu IC, Lin CC, Hsiung CA, et al. Epidemiology of sarcopenia among community-dwelling older adults in Taiwan: a pooled analysis for a broader adoption of sarcopenia assessments. Geriatr Gerontol Int 2014;1:52–60.
11. Abate M, Di Iorio A, Di Renzo D, et al. Frailty in the elderly: the physical dimension. Europa Medicophys 2007;43(3):407–15.
12. Faulkner JA, Larkin LM, Claflin DR, et al. Age-related changes in the structure and function of skeletal muscles. Clin Exp Pharmacol Physiol 2007;34(11):1091–6.
13. Ryall JG, Schertzer JD, Lynch GS. Cellular and molecular mechanisms underlying age-related skeletal muscle wasting and weakness. Biogerontology 2008;9(4):213–28.
14. Marcell TJ. Sarcopenia: causes, consequences, and preventions. J Gerontol A Biol Sci Med Sci 2003;58(10):M911–6.
15. Booth FW, Chakravarthy MV, Spangenburg EE. Exercise and gene expression: physiological regulation of the human genome through physical activity. J Physiol 2002;543(Pt 2):399–411.
16. Sayer AA, Syddall HE, Gilbody HJ, et al. Does sarcopenia originate in early life? Findings from the Hertfordshire cohort study. J Gerontol A Biol Sci Med Sci 2004;59(9):M930–4.

17. Sayer AA, Dennison EM, Syddall HE, et al. The developmental origins of sarcopenia: using peripheral quantitative computed tomography to assess muscle size in older people. J Gerontol A Biol Sci Med Sci 2008;63(8):835–40.
18. Patel HP, Jameson KA, Syddall HE, et al. Developmental influences, muscle morphology, and sarcopenia in community-dwelling older men. J Gerontol A Biol Sci Med Sci 2012;67(1):82–7.
19. Cesari M, Fielding RA, Pahor M, et al. Biomarkers of sarcopenia in clinical trials-recommendations from the International Working Group on sarcopenia. J Cachexia Sarcopenia Muscle 2012;3(3):181–90.
20. Abellan van Kan G, Cderbaum JM, Cesari M, et al. Sarcopenia: biomarkers and imaging (international conference on sarcopenia research). J Nutr Health Aging 2011;15(10):834–46.
21. Muscaritoli M, Anker SD, Argiles J, et al. Consensus definition of sarcopenia, cachexia and pre-cachexia: joint document elaborated by Special Interest Groups (SIG) "cachexia-anorexia in chronic wasting diseases" and "nutrition in geriatrics". Clin Nutr 2010;29(2):154–9.
22. Abellan van Kan G, Houles M, Vellas B. Identifying sarcopenia. Curr Opin Clin Nutr Metab Care 2012;15(5):436–41.
23. Doherty TJ. Invited review: aging and sarcopenia. J Appl Physiol (1985) 2003; 95(4):1717–27.
24. Lexell J, Taylor CC, Sjostrom M. What is the cause of the ageing atrophy? Total number, size and proportion of different fiber types studied in whole vastus lateralis muscle from 15- to 83-year-old men. J Neurol Sci 1988;84(2–3):275–94.
25. Doherty TJ, Brown WF. Age-related changes in the twitch contractile properties of human thenar motor units. J Appl Physiol 1985;82(1):93–101.
26. Tomlinson BE, Irving D. The numbers of limb motor neurons in the human lumbosacral cord throughout life. J Neurol Sci 1977;34(2):213–9.
27. Yarasheski KE. Exercise, aging, and muscle protein metabolism. J Gerontol A Biol Sci Med Sci 2003;58(10):M918–22.
28. Roth SM, Ferrell RF, Hurley BF. Strength training for the prevention and treatment of sarcopenia. J Nutr Health Aging 2000;4(3):143–55.
29. Denison HJ, Cooper C, Sayer AA, et al. Prevention and optimal management of sarcopenia: a review of combined exercise and nutrition interventions to improve muscle outcomes in older people. Clin Interv Aging 2015;10:859–69.
30. Sakuma K, Yamaguchi A. Sarcopenia and age-related endocrine function. Int J Endocrinol 2012;2012:127362.
31. Wakabayashi H, Sakuma K. Comprehensive approach to sarcopenia treatment. Curr Clin Pharmacol 2014;9(2):171–80.
32. Lynch GS. Emerging drugs for sarcopenia: age-related muscle wasting. Expert Opin Emerg Drugs 2004;9(2):345–61.
33. Dingemans AM, de Vos-Geelen J, Langen R, et al. Phase II drugs that are currently in development for the treatment of cachexia. Expert Opin Investig Drugs 2014;23(12):1655–69.
34. Stewart Coats AJ, Srinivasan V, Surendran J, et al. The ACT-ONE trial, a multicentre, randomised, double-blind, placebo-controlled, dose-finding study of the anabolic/catabolic transforming agent, MT-102 in subjects with cachexia related to stage III and IV non-small cell lung cancer and colorectal cancer: study design. J Cachexia Sarcopenia Muscle 2011;2(4):201–7.
35. Potsch MS, Tschirner A, Palus S, et al. The anabolic catabolic transforming agent (ACTA) espindolol increases muscle mass and decreases fat mass in old rats.

J Cachexia Sarcopenia Muscle 2014;5(2):149–58. Available at: http://www.ncbi.nlm.nih.gov/pubmed/24272787.

36. Molfino A, Amabile MI, Rossi Fanelli F, et al. Novel therapeutic options for cachexia and sarcopenia. Expert Opin Biol Ther 2016;16(10):1239–44.

37. Rondanelli M, Miccono A, Peroni G, et al. A systematic review on the effects of botanicals on skeletal muscle health in order to prevent sarcopenia. Evid Based Complement Alternat Med 2016;5970367(10):9.

38. Konishi M, Ishida J, von Haehling S, et al. Nutrition in cachexia: from bench to bedside. J Cachexia Sarcopenia Muscle 2016;7(2):107–9.

39. Relph WL. Addressing the nutritional needs of older patients. Nurs Older People 2016;28(3):16–9.

40. Phillips SM, Chevalier S, Leidy HJ. Protein "requirements" beyond the RDA: implications for optimizing health. Appl Physiol Nutr Metab 2016;9:1–8.

41. Thomas DR. Loss of skeletal muscle mass in aging: examining the relationship of starvation, sarcopenia and cachexia. Clin Nutr 2007;26(4):389–99.

42. Evans WJ, Morley JE, Argiles J, et al. Cachexia: a new definition. Clin Nutr 2008;27(6):793–9.

43. Morley JE, Anker SD, Evans WJ. Cachexia and aging: an update based on the fourth international cachexia meeting. J Nutr Health Aging 2009;13(1):47–55.

44. Durham WJ, Dillon EL, Sheffield-Moore M. Inflammatory burden and amino acid metabolism in cancer cachexia. Curr Opin Clin Nutr Metab Care 2009;12(1):72–7.

45. Bauer JM, Kaiser MJ, Sieber CC. Sarcopenia in nursing home residents. J Am Med Dir Assoc 2008;9(8):545–51.

46. Fried LP, Tangen CM, Walston J, et al. Frailty in older adults: evidence for a phenotype. J Gerontol A Biol Sci Med Sci 2001;56(3):M146–56.

47. Prado CM, Lieffers JR, McCargar LJ, et al. Prevalence and clinical implications of sarcopenic obesity in patients with solid tumours of the respiratory and gastrointestinal tracts: a population-based study. Lancet Oncol 2008;9(7):629–35.

48. Waters DL, Baumgartner RN. Sarcopenia and obesity. Clin Geriatr Med 2011;27(3):401–21.

49. Stenholm S, Harris TB, Rantanen T, et al. Sarcopenic obesity: definition, cause and consequences. Curr Opin Clin Nutr Metab Care 2008;11(6):693–700.

50. Ding J, Kritchevsky SB, Newman AB, et al. Effects of birth cohort and age on body composition in a sample of community-based elderly. Am J Clin Nutr 2007;85(2):405–10.

51. Song MY, Ruts E, Kim J, et al. Sarcopenia and increased adipose tissue infiltration of muscle in elderly African American women. Am J Clin Nutr 2004;79(5):874–80.

52. Hughes VA, Roubenoff R, Wood M, et al. Anthropometric assessment of 10-y changes in body composition in the elderly. Am J Clin Nutr 2004;80(2):475–82.

53. Morley JE. Sarcopenia: diagnosis and treatment. J Nutr Health Aging 2008;12(7):452–6.

54. Beard JR, Officer AM, Cassels AK. The world report on ageing and health. Gerontologist 2016;56(Suppl 2):S163–6.

55. Sayer AA. Sarcopenia the new geriatric giant: time to translate research findings into clinical practice. Age Ageing 2014;43(6):736–7.

56. Sayer AA. Sarcopenia. BMJ 2010;341:c4097.

57. Sayer AA, Robinson SM, Patel HP, et al. New horizons in the pathogenesis, diagnosis and management of sarcopenia. Age Ageing 2013;42(2):145–50.

A Review of Osteoporosis in the Older Adult

Paloma Alejandro, MD*, Florina Constantinescu, MD, MS, PhD

KEYWORDS

- Osteoporosis • Bisphosphonates • FRAX • Drug holiday • Hip fractures • Elderly
- DXA

KEY POINTS

- Fractures and osteoporosis are common, especially in the elderly population. Hip fractures may be devastating.
- Osteoporosis in men is greatly unrecognized and untreated.
- Treatment of osteoporosis is generally recommended in postmenopausal women and men 50 years old or older who have a bone mineral density T score of −2.5 or less, a history of previous spine or hip fracture, or a Fracture Risk Assessment Tool score indicating increased fracture risk.
- Bisphosphonates, teriparatide and denosumab have proven to reduce risk of hip, vertebral, and nonvertebral fractures. Bisphosphonates are used usually as first-line treatment in patients if no contraindications. Teriparatide reduces the risk of nonvertebral and vertebral fractures.
- Individualizing therapy is important. This includes balancing the risks and benefits of bisphosphonates in order to enact a drug holiday. For patients at lower risk for fracture, drug holidays after 5 years of alendronate therapy or 3 years of zoledronic acid therapy can be considered.

INTRODUCTION

Osteoporosis is a disorder with major impact in Western society and globally, and osteoporotic fractures are associated with significant burden of health care cost, morbidity, and mortality.[1] A vast majority of patients remain undiagnosed and untreated, especially high-risk patients.[2] In patients 65 years and older, the increase in incidence of osteoporotic fractures is accompanied by grim effects on disability and mortality.[3] Older patients are at increased risk of nursing home admissions and long-term stay after hip osteoporotic fractures, as compared with myocardial infarctions and stroke.[4] In 2014, a discouraging study was published assessing the frequency of starting bisphosphonate treatment after hip fracture in the United States

Disclosure Statement: The authors have nothing to disclose.
Division of Rheumatology, MedStar Washington Hospital Center, Georgetown University Medical Center, 110 Irving Street Northwest 2A-66, Washington, DC 20010, USA
* Corresponding author.
E-mail address: paloma.alejandro@medstar.net

Clin Geriatr Med 33 (2017) 27–40
http://dx.doi.org/10.1016/j.cger.2016.08.003
0749-0690/17/© 2016 Elsevier Inc. All rights reserved.
geriatric.theclinics.com

(2002–2011). In 2002, 40% of the patients started medication within 12 months of hip fracture, which decreased to less than 20% in 2011 nationwide.[5]

Osteoporosis is defined as a deterioration in bone mass and microarchitecture of bone, along with increased fragility, that predisposes bones to fracture.[6] Two main pathophysiologic processes generate bone loss. The first results from estrogen deficiency and affects trabecular bone, known as postmenopausal osteoporosis. This type of osteoporosis affects mainly women and is associated with vertebral fractures and hip fractures. Osteoblasts respond to many external and internal stimuli including hormones (parathyroid hormone [PTH], vitamin D). As a result to these stimuli, macrophage colony-stimulating factor and membrane-bound receptor activator of nuclear factor-kappa B ligand (RANKL) are produced. These, in turn, are critical factors for osteoclastogenesis. Binding of RANKL with its receptor RANK in osteoclasts stimulates their differentiation and prevents osteoclast cell death. Osteoprotegerin produced by osteoblasts inhibits the RANK-RANKL pathway.[7] Conversely, estrogen, transforming growth factor-β, and mechanical force inhibit RANKL expression, thus suppressing osteoclast cell formation and differentiation, ultimately decreasing bone resorption.[8]

Another advance in bone biology is the Wnt (wingless-type MMTV integration site) signaling pathway in osteoblasts, which is important for bone formation. Inhibitors of this pathway are sclerostin and dick-kopf WNT signaling pathway inhibitor 1. Sclerostin is expressed in osteocytes as a response to mechanical stress.[9]

A second type, recently known as senile osteoporosis, mainly affects cortical bone, predisposing elderly patients to hip fractures. These changes in bone mass associated with aging are multifactorial; they include changes in hormones as well as vitamin D insufficiency, leading to secondary hyperparathyroidism, thereby enhancing osteoclastic bone resorption. Recent evidence of a possible link between aging and senile osteoporosis has been described. Lack of lamin A/C, a special scaffolding protein found in bone structure cells, is seen in aging osteoblasts and is associated with reduced osteoblastic activity, lipodystrophy, and fat redistribution as observed in mice studies.[10]

Osteoporosis in men may be secondary to hypogonadism, corticosteroid use, and excessive alcohol use. In men, bone loss increases after age 70. Osteoporosis in men remains untreated and unrecognized.[11,12] In a study of elderly male nursing home residents with hip fractures, 66% of the patients had hypogonadism.[13] In elderly male patients, vertebral fractures are more common.[14] Testosterone depletion has direct effects on cortical and trabecular bone mass resulting in decreased bone mineral density (BMD) in hypogonadal patients.[15] Osteoporosis is most often identified after the first hip fracture, which itself is a risk factor for future osteoporotic fractures.[11]

A comprehensive approach to the diagnosis and management of osteoporosis includes a detailed history, physical examination, BMD assessment, radiological studies to diagnose fractures, and FRAX World Health Organization (WHO) 10 year estimated fracture probability calculation. The diagnosis of osteoporosis by WHO criteria is established by BMD measurement using dual-energy x-ray absorptiometry (DXA) scanning or by adult vertebral or hip fracture in the absence of major trauma.[16] DXA measurement of the hip and spine is used to establish and confirm the diagnosis of osteoporosis. The BMD predicts fracture risk and has been shown to correlate with bone strength and future fracture risk.[16] BMD is expressed in grams per square centimeters, and it is compared with an adult population of the same gender (T score), or to the BMD of an age-, sex-, and ethnicity-matched reference population (Z score). Osteoporosis and low bone mass have been defined based on DXA measurements (**Table 1**).

Table 1
Osteoporosis and low bone mass based on bone mineral density measurement by dual-energy x-ray absorptiometry

Category	Bone Mass Measurement
Normal	T score greater than or equal to −1 SD
Osteopenia	T score less than −1 and greater than −2.5 SD
Osteoporosis	T score less than or equal to −2.5 SD
Severe osteoporosis	T score greater than than −2.5 in the presence of fracture

Abbreviation: SD, standard deviation.
Data from WHO scientific group on the assessment of osteoporosis at the primary health care level: summary meeting report, 2004. Geneva (Switzerland): World Health Organization; 2007.

The National Osteoporosis Foundation (NOF) has established screening guidelines for osteoporosis. Routine screening with DXA should be performed in women aged 65 or older and postmenopausal women less than 65 years old based on risk factors. Screening should also be done in men older than 70 years old and men between 50 and 69 years old based on risk factors.[17]

Vertebral imaging should be performed for surveillance of subclinical osteoporotic fractures in all women aged 70 and older and all men 80 and older if BMD T score is less than or equal to −1.5 at the spine, total hip, or femoral neck in order to treat fractures and decrease mortality in this population of patients. In postmenopausal women and men aged 50 and older with risk factors like historical height loss, low-trauma fracture, or prospective height loss, long-term corticosteroid treatment performing vertebral imaging is also recommended.[16] Laboratory testing is recommended to exclude secondary causes like multiple myeloma, gastrointestinal malabsorption, diabetes mellitus, primary hyperparathyroidism, inflammatory bowel disease, ankylosing spondylitis, and rheumatoid arthritis, among others. As part of the evaluation, a calcium and vitamin D level evaluation should be done.

The WHO Fracture Risk Assessment Tool (FRAX) score is used to estimate fracture risk in patients (https://www.shef.ac.uk/FRAX/tool). This tool applies to patients with low femoral neck BMD, between ages 40 and 90 years old. FRAX can be calculated with either femoral neck or total hip, but when available, femoral neck is preferred.[18] FRAX is to be evaluated alongside clinical risk factors for fractures and can be used for both sexes (**Box 1**).

Osteoporosis treatment should be initiated in those patients with hip or vertebral fractures, asymptomatic or clinical, in those patients with T scores less than or equal to −2.5 at the femoral neck, total hip, or lumbar spine by DXA, in postmenopausal women and men aged 50 and older with low bone mass (T score between −1.0 and −2.5, osteopenia) at the femoral neck, total hip, or lumbar spine by DXA and a 10-year hip fracture probability equal to or greater than 3% or a 10-year major osteoporosis-related fracture probability equal or greater than 20% based on the US-adapted WHO FRAX model (**Box 2**).[16,19]

There are several caveats when using this tool, and clinical judgment must be used. In patients with low BMD in the lumbar spine but a normal femoral neck BMD, using FRAX tool tends to underestimate fracture risk. FRAX also can underestimate risk of fracture in patients with diabetes mellitus, which confers increased risk of fracture independent of FRAX-derived assessment with the BMD.[20] It has not been validated to be used in patients on current or previous osteoporosis treatment. Finally, patients

---

Box 1
Clinical risk factors for fractures included in Fracture Risk Assessment Tool

- History of smoking
- Alcohol abuse
- History of rheumatoid arthritis
- Secondary osteoporosis (inflammatory bowel disease, premature menopause, hypogonadism, chronic liver disease, malabsorption syndromes)
- Advanced age
- History of fractures
- History of glucocorticoid treatment
- Family history of hip fracture, parental
- Low body weight

Data from Kanis JA, Borgstrom F, De Laet C, et al. Assessment of fracture risk. Osteoporos Int 2005;16:581.

---

who have been on a drug holiday for 1 to 2 years may be considered as untreated patients when using this tool.[21]

In terms of treatment options for osteoporosis, the NOF recommends starting with a nonpharmacologic approach. Resistance and weight-bearing exercise can increase muscle mass and transiently increase BMD.[22] Tai chi and yoga improve balance and increase muscle tone, which as a secondary effect reduces the risk for falls among elderly patients. Counseling about smoking cessation (which is directly linked to reduced BMD) and alcohol cessation are encouraged.[23] However, the efficacy of calcium and vitamin D treatment remains a controversial topic. Vitamin D supplementation has not been shown across the board to reduce the risk of fractures or to increase the BMD.[24] Meta-analyses of several large trials of calcium and vitamin D supplementation given separately were ineffective preventing hip fracture. Given in combination, calcium and vitamin D was associated with an absolute risk reduction of 0.5% over 3 years, corresponding to a number needed to treat of 213 people treated for 3 years to prevent a hip fracture. For patients greater than the age of 70, the absolute risk reduction was 0.9%.[25] In the Women's Health Initiative trial, women assigned to

---

Box 2
Guidelines for treatment of osteoporosis

History of hip or vertebral fracture

T score greater than or equal to −2.5 (DXA) at the femoral neck or spine

T score between −1 and −2.5 at the femoral neck or spine, and a 10-year probability of hip fracture ≥3% or a 10-year probability of any major osteoporosis-related fracture ≥20% based on the US -adapted FRAX algorithm

Data from Cosman F, de Beur SJ, LeBoff MS, et al. Clinician's guide to prevention and treatment of osteoporosis. Osteoporos Int 2014;25:2359; and Watts NB, Adler RA, Bilezikian JP, et al. Osteoporosis in men: an Endocrine Society clinical practice guideline. J Clin Endocrinol Metab 2012;97:1802.

take calcium and vitamin D had an increase in BMD and a decrease by 12% in hip fracture compared to women assigned to placebo. There were no significant reductions in clinical vertebral fracture, fracture of the lower arm or wrist, or total fractures, but had a 17% higher risk of developing kidney stones compared with placebo. The mean calcium intake was approximately 1150 mg per day.[26] The NOF recommends men aged 50 to 70 consume 1000 mg per day of calcium and women aged 51 and older and men aged 71 and older consume 1200 mg per day of calcium. In terms of vitamin D supplementation, NOF recommends an intake of 800 to 1000 international units (IU) of vitamin D per day for adults aged 50 and older. At present, reasonable recommendations for postmenopausal women and men with osteoporosis is 1000 to 1500 mg per day of calcium and 600 to 800 IU per day of vitamin D.[16]

In a study by Amory and colleagues,[27] testosterone therapy with finasteride was used as treatment in older men with low serum testosterone levels (<200 ng/dL). After 3 years, an increase in BMD in the lumbar spine was observed. Finasteride also helped to decrease the prostate growth and PSA levels. Testosterone therapy is also controversial. Its side effects may be detrimental because it can cause polycythemia, sleep apnea, and prostate cancer. Additional data are needed in order to safely use this agent in eugonadal men.

Pharmacologic therapies can be classified as antiresorptive, targeting osteoclast-mediated bone resorption, or anabolic, targeting stimulation of osteoblasts for new bone formation. Selective estrogen-receptor modulators (SERMs) activate tissue receptors for estrogen. Raloxifene is an SERM approved by the US Food and Drug Adminstration to treat osteoporosis. It inhibits bone resorption, increases spine BMD, and decreases vertebral fractures, but has no effect on nonvertebral or hip fractures.[28] Raloxifene decreases the risk of breast cancer among high-risk patients but increases thromboembolic events.[29]

Bisphosphonates inhibit bone remodeling, and both oral and intravenous (IV) forms have been shown in randomized trials to reduce risk of fractures. Side effects include gastric ulcers and reflux, and they should not be prescribed in patients with clinical significant esophageal disease, such as achalasia. In two Fracture Intervention Trials of Alendronate, paired randomized trials, with 3 to 4 years follow-up involving postmenopausal women with a BMD T score of -1.6 or less at the femoral neck, the rate of vertebral fractures was significantly lower by 50% among those who received alendronate compared with placebo.[30,31] Black and colleagues[30] studied women aged 55 to 81 with low-femoral neck BMD and at least one vertebral fracture at baseline and enrolled them in 2 study groups based on presence or absence of an existing vertebral fracture. Women were randomly assigned to placebo or alendronate and followed up for 36 months. They found that among women with low bone mass and existing vertebral fractures, alendronate reduced the frequency of morphometric (radiological) and clinical vertebral fractures. In the second trial, Cummings and colleagues[31] evaluated women in the Fracture Intervention Trial without existing vertebral fractures. Women aged 54 to 81 years old with a femoral neck BMD of 0.68 g/cm^2 or less, but no vertebral fracture, were randomized to alendronate or placebo for 4 years. In women with low BMD but without vertebral fractures, 4 years of alendronate safely increased BMD and decreased the risk of first vertebral fracture. Alendronate significantly reduced the risk of clinical fractures among women with osteoporosis at femoral neck by 36% but not among women with higher BMD. Alendronate decreased the risk of radiographic vertebral fractures by 44% overall (number needed to treat, 60).

Two randomized controlled trials for risedronate are important: VERT-NA and VERT-MN trials. Harris and colleagues[32] (the VERT-NA trial) studied postmenopausal women with existing vertebral fractures, low BMD in the spine, or both. Over a period of 3 years, the risk of fractures was lower by 49% with risedronate than placebo. A significant reduction was observed in the risk of new vertebral fractures by 65% and 61% after the first year of treatment with risedronate in VERT-NA and VERT-MN studies, respectively. This effect was maintained throughout the 3 years of treatment with significant reduction in the incidence of new vertebral fractures by 41% in VERT-NA and by 49% in VERT-MN. In VERT-NA, the risk of fractures in the first year of treatment in patients with at least 2 or more vertebral fractures was 74%. Risedronate also significantly reduced the risk of nonvertebral fractures by 39% after 3 years in VERT-NA.[33] McClung and colleagues[34] studied the endpoint of hip fracture in the Hip Intervention Program. Risedronate (2.5 mg or 5 mg a day) was given to women 70 years or older who were at high risk for hip fracture; they showed a 30% reduction rate of hip fractures over 3 years as compared with placebo.

Chestnut and colleagues[35] studied ibandronate in a 3-year multicenter antifracture study. Patients were randomized to treatment with either continuous oral ibandronate (2.5 mg daily), intermittent oral ibandronate (20 mg every other day for 12 doses every 3 months), or placebo. A 62% lower rate of vertebral fractures was observed compared with placebo, but no reduction in rate of nonvertebral fractures was seen over a period of 3 years. Later, in the MOBILE Study, the efficacy and safety of once-monthly ibandronate with daily ibandronate was compared. Substantial increases in lumbar spine BMD were seen in all treatment arms in the daily and once-monthly groups. It was confirmed that all once-monthly regimens were at least as effective as daily treatment. Substantial increases in total hip, femoral neck, and trochanter BMD were seen; the dose of 150 mg produced the most pronounced effect ($P<.05$ vs daily treatment). Independent of the regimen, most patients (70.5%–93.5%) achieved increases above baseline in lumbar spine or total hip BMD or both.[36] This medication is also available as an IV and can be used when oral bisphosphonates are not well tolerated. In the DIVA study, the optimal ibandronate IV injection schedule for the treatment of postmenopausal osteoporosis was studied, comparing the efficacy and tolerability of 2- and 3-monthly injections with the previously evaluated daily oral ibandronate regimen.[37] Postmenopausal women aged 55 to 80 years old with osteoporosis (mean lumbar spine BMD T score <-2.5 or worse) were included. At 2 years, the 2- and 3-monthly IV regimens achieved statistical noninferiority and also superior increases in lumbar spine BMD compared with the daily regimen. Greater increases were also obtained with IV ibandronate versus daily oral in proximal femur BMD.[37]

In a large randomized controlled trial (HORIZON-PFT) in women with low BMD or with vertebral fractures, or both, a once per year infusion of zoledronic acid 5 mg resulted in significantly low rates of vertebral fractures by 70%, hip fractures by 41%, and nonvertebral fractures by 25%.[38] Because zoledronic acid can cause an acute-phase reaction (flulike symptoms up to 3 days after infusion), coadministration of acetaminophen may be used to reduce the incidence and severity of these side effects.[39] In the metanalysis of Minyan and colleagues, zolendronic acid was shown to be effective in the prevention of vertebral and nonvertebral fractures as well as in increasing the BMD.[40]

In terms of biological agents, denosumab was the first biologic introduced for osteoporosis treatment. It is a fully human monoclonal RANKL antibody. It prevents binding of RANKL to RANK, leading to inhibition of osteoclast activation. In the FREEDOM trial, postmenopausal women aged 60 to 90 years old with a lumbar spine or total hip BMD T score less than −2.5 but no less than −4.0 at the lumbar spine or total hip were randomized to receive placebo or denosumab 60 mg, administered subcutaneously every 6 months. Denosumab significantly reduced vertebral fractures, hip fractures, and nonvertebral fractures, with a cumulative incidence of 2.3% in the denosumab group versus 7.2% in the placebo group (relative risk 0.32) for vertebral fractures. In terms of risk of hip fracture, in the denosumab group a cumulative incidence of 0.7% versus 1.2% in the placebo group was observed. For nonvertebral fractures, the cumulative incidence for denosumab treatment was 6.5% versus 8.0% in the placebo group.[41] In the FREEDOM extension trial, the effects of denosumab on bone mass over the long term were studied. This study captured up to 8 years of denosumab exposure for women who received 3 years of denosumab in FREEDOM and then continued in the extension (long-term group), and up to 5 years of denosumab exposure for women who received 3 years of placebo in FREEDOM and then transitioned to denosumab in the extension (crossover group). In the long-term group, mean BMD continued to increase for cumulative 8-year gains of 18.4% and 8.3% at the lumbar spine and total hip, respectively. In the crossover group, the mean BMD increased significantly from the extension baseline for 5-year cumulative gains of 13.1% and 6.2% at the lumbar spine and total hip, respectively. The yearly incidence of new vertebral and nonvertebral fractures remained low in both groups. Denosumab treatment for up to 8 years was associated with continued BMD gains, low fracture incidence, and a consistent safety profile.[42]

Miller and colleagues[43] assessed the long-term efficacy and the effects of discontinuing and restarting denosumab in postmenopausal women with low bone mass. They observed that the effects on bone turnover were fully reversible with discontinuation of denosumab and later restored after re-treatment. There is a possibility of that denosumab in combination with other biologics agents could increase the risk for infections because RANK-RANKL are members of the tumor necrosis factor (TNF)/TNF receptor superfamilies.[44]

In the anabolic family of medications teriparatide can be found, which is a parathyroid hormone analogue. It is the first anabolic medication approved to treat osteoporosis. Continuous PTH has catabolic effects, whereas daily intermittent PTH has anabolic skeletal effects.[45] Teriparatide was studied in women with previous vertebral fractures. It was associated with decreased vertebral and nonvertebral fractures as compared with placebo.[46] Teriparatide is useful in reducing vertebral fractures risk in patients with prior vertebral fractures. It can also be used in patients with severe osteoporosis in which rapid bone growth is needed. Following a course of teriparatide, which can be given for a maximum of 2 years as recommended by the NOF, antiresorptives should be used to preserve or increase gain in BMD acquired by teriparatide.[47] Sequential treatment with teriparatide and denosumab resulted in a greater increase in BMD compared with switching of therapy.[48]

The main reasons to consider a drug holiday and limit the use of bisphosphonates are possible adverse effects such as osteonecrosis of the jaw and atypical femoral fractures. Osteonecrosis of the jaw is defined as the presence of exposed and necrotic bone in the maxillofacial bone that does not heal within 8 weeks. In patients who may undergo invasive dental procedures, mainly tooth extractions, bisphosphonates may increase the risk of osteonecrosis of the jaw. Recently, it has been described that the patients at highest risk of developing this complication are those with malignancy-related skeletal conditions receiving high doses of IV bisphosphonates. The risk is proportional to the duration and cumulative dose of bisphosphonates; it is very rare, and the estimated incidence rate is less than 1:10,000 patient-years.[49] A recent review suggests that before major invasive dental surgery, consideration should be given to stopping bisphosphonate therapy. It appears that good dental hygiene reduces the risk.[50]

Another feared complication is atypical femur fractures. In all case controlled randomized trials and cohort studies that have studied the relationship of atypical femur fracture and bisphosphonate treatment, the incidence of these fractures remains low.[51,52] Studies have suggested that there is an increased risk after more than 5 years of bisphosphonate use.[53,54] Numerically, these fractures account for 4 to 5 of every 1000 femur fractures reported.[52]

A major criterion for atypical femur fractures is a fracture below the lesser trochanter of the femur. The main prodromal symptom is unilateral or bilateral dull or aching pain in the groin or thigh. A cohort study in Kaiser California examined 142 atypical fractures and found that 128 of those patients were on bisphosphonates; this was observed 1 to 2 years into treatment, and the incidence was 1.8/100,000/patient-years. After more than 8 years, the incidence increased to 113/100,000/patient-year.[55] The incidence of typical femur fractures (femoral neck and trochanteric fractures) is of 750 to 833/100,000/patient-years after 8 years of treatment. For evaluation of suspected atypical femoral fracture, radiograph, bone scan, or MRI is indicated. It has been shown that 25% of the cases involve bilateral hips. In some case reports, patients with atypical femur fractures have been treated with teriparatide.[56]

Studies of bisphosphonates and the risk of atypical femur fractures with bisphosphonate use at 3 years have described a relative risk of 47.3 with both alendronate and risedronate.[57] Upon discontinuing any of the bisphosphonates, after 1 year, the relative risk of fracture decreases significantly to 3.5.

Therefore careful consideration by the physician of the risk of hip fracture and benefits/risks of bisphosphonates is necessary. For example, it has been argued that a patient with a T score of −3.0 and a vertebral fracture in the last 2 years may not be an optimal candidate for discontinuation of therapy.[58–60]

Studies have shown that bisphosphonates may have a long-term residual effect on bone mass. Rodan and colleagues[61] described that after 10 years of alendronate therapy, and during a drug holiday, the medication will continue to be present in detectable levels. This finding raises the question about which patients will continue to have a benefit during greater than 5 years of bisphosphonate treatment. In the FLEX long-term extension trial, patients were randomized to alendronate, 5 mg/d, 10 mg/d, or placebo. After 5 years of treatment, the cumulative risk of nonvertebral fractures was not significantly different between those continuing (19%) and discontinuing (18.9%) alendronate. Among those who continued, there was a significantly lower risk of clinically recognized vertebral fractures (5.3% for placebo and 2.4% for alendronate), but no significant reduction in morphometric vertebral fractures, which are fractures seen radiologically (11.3% for placebo and 9.8% for alendronate).[58] Bauer and colleagues[62] studied methods of predicting fracture risk in the FLEX study among women who have discontinued alendronate after 5 years. During 5 years of placebo, 94 of 437 women (22%) experienced 1 or more symptomatic fractures and 82 had fractures after 1 year. The 1-year changes in hip DXA were not related to subsequent fracture risk, but older age and lower hip DXA at time of discontinuation were significantly related to increased fracture risk (total hip DXA relative hazard ratio, 1.87) In a post hoc analysis of FLEX, Schwartz and colleagues[63] evaluated postmenopausal women originally randomized to alendronate in the FIT trial who were treated for 5 years. Patients were randomized to placebo (40%) or alendronate 5 mg/d (30%) or alendronate 10 mg/d (30%) for an additional 5 years. Among women without vertebral fracture at FLEX baseline, continuation of alendronate reduced nonvertebral fractures in women with femoral neck T scores of −2.5 or worse but not with T scores greater than −2.5 or better. Continuing alendronate for 10 years, instead of stopping after 5 years, reduces nonvertebral risk in women without prevalent vertebral fracture whose femoral neck T scores after 5 years of alendronate are −2.5 or worse but does not reduce risk of nonvertebral fracture in women whose T scores are −2 or better.

In the HORIZON-PFT extension trial, zoledronic acid at 6 years is compared with zoledronic acid at 3 years. In this study, postmenopausal women who received zoledronic acid for 3 years in HORIZON were randomized to 3 additional years of zoledronic acid or placebo. The primary endpoint was femoral neck BMD percentage change from year 3 to 6 in the intend-to-treat population. In years 3 to 6, femoral neck BMD remained constant in the zoledronic acid group and dropped slightly in the placebo group (but nevertheless remained greater than pretreatment levels). Other BMD sites showed similar differences. New vertebral fractures were lower in the zoledronic acid group at 6 years versus placebo, whereas other fractures were not different. In conclusion, this study demonstrated that fracture reductions suggest that those at high fracture risk, particularly vertebral fracture, may benefit from continued treatment.[59,60] Subsequently, Black and colleagues[60] studied a second extension to 9 years of zoledronic acid in the HORIZON-PFT. In this study, women on zoledronic acid for 6 years in the first extension were randomized to either zoledronic acid or placebo for 3 additional years. The primary endpoint was change in total hip BMD at year 9 versus placebo. From year 6 to 9, the mean change in total hip BMD was −0.54% in the 3 additional years of zoledronic acid versus −1.31% in placebo group. The number of fractures was low and did not significantly differ by treatment. The results suggest almost all patients who have received 6 annual zoledronic acid infusions can stop medication for up to 3 years with apparent maintenance of benefits. A post hoc analysis by Cosman and colleagues[64] using HORIZON trial data sought to define significant predictors of fracture and attempted to quantify fracture incidence in risk factor-defined subgroups of women who discontinued zoledronic acid after 3 years of treatment. Fracture risk after 6 years of zoledronic acid versus 3 years of zoledronic acid versus placebo was studied. They showed that patients with a T score of −2.5 or worse were more likely to have morphometric vertebral fractures on placebo versus zoledronic acid. After 3 years of zoledronic acid (in women with a total hip T score greater than −2.5, no recent incident fracture and no more than one risk factor), the risk for subsequent fracture over 3 additional years remains low for morphometric vertebral fracture if treatment is discontinued (vertebral fracture, average risk 3.2%, and for nonvertebral fracture, average risk 5.8%). In these patients, discontinuation for up to 3 years is therefore reasonable. No difference for patients with osteopenia was observed as to the incidence of vertebral fractures, implying that this population can safely undergo a drug holiday.

In another post hoc analysis, Reid and colleagues[65] analyzed patients on HORIZON-PFT trial. They observed that the rate of reduction in fracture after 1 year of zoledronic acid compared with 3 years of zoledronic acid uncovered a 32% reduction in clinical fracture as compared with 34% in 3 years. Because this study suggests no significant difference of fracture risk reduction at 1 year and 3 years, then a single infusion of zoledronic acid may be sufficient to reduce the risk of fracture. Larger studies will be needed to confirm this finding.

Black and colleagues[21] concluded that patients with low BMD at the femoral neck (T score below −2.5) despite 3 to 5 years of treatment are at highest risk for vertebral fractures and therefore appear to benefit most from continuation of bisphosphonates.

Patients with an existing vertebral fracture who have a T score at −2.0 may also benefit from continued therapy. Patients with a femoral neck T score greater than −2.0 have a low risk of vertebral fracture and are unlikely to benefit from continued treatment.[21] These recommendations might change as additional data regarding long-term therapy with bisphosphonates becomes available.

A review of the literature as provided here suggests that a rational therapeutic approach should include assessment if treatment with oral bisphosphonates is needed for more than 5 years in those patients who have a low hip T score of less or equal to −2.5 at 5 years of alendronate therapy and at 3 years of zolendronate therapy. Extension of treatment in those patients 75 years old or older, who have a history of vertebral fractures during therapy, may require specialty consultation.[21]

During a drug holiday, patients may be reassessed every 2 to 3 years by DXA. Therapy can be restarted in patients who have a new clinical fracture. However, it is possible that a drug holiday may be longer for patients exposed to zoledronic acid or alendronate as compared with risedronate/ibandronate due to differences in bone binding affinity of the medications.

In the recent years, and thanks to new advances in knowledge of bone biology, new therapies have emerged, specific to different pathways of the bone-remodeling schema. Abaloparatide is a human recombinant-related PTH hormone, which is given by daily subcutaneous injection. This medication binds to PTH 1 receptor, resulting in lower bone resorption, less hypercalcemia, and less cortical porosity.[66] Leder and colleagues[66] studied abaloparatide, comparing it with teriparatide and placebo in postmenopausal women. As compared with placebo, 24 weeks of daily subcutaneous abaloparatide increases BMD of the lumbar spine, femoral neck, and total hip in a dose-dependent fashion. Abaloparatide increases in BMD at the total hip are greater than with teriparatide. Hypercalcemia in a 4-hour infusion was less. Also, active trials comparing abaloparatide to teriparatide have shown no significant difference between the two medications in terms of nonvertebral and vertebral fractures. Results of the phase 3 pivotal fracture trial with abaloparatide were recently presented.[67] In more than 18 months of treatment with abaloparatide and teriparatide, the incidence of vertebral fracture was decreased by 86% and 80%, respectively, compared with placebo. A significant 43% reduction in nonvertebral fracture risk was observed with abaloparatide. The difference in nonvertebral risk reduction between abaloparatide and teriparatide was not significant.

Other medications receiving attention in the past year are the humanized monoclonal antibodies against sclerostin, romosozumab, and blosozumab, which decrease bone resorption. In a phase 2 trial of postmenopausal women, romosozumab was found to be superior to teriparatide and alendronate in increasing BMD in spine, total hip, and femoral neck.[68] Increase in bone mass density was 11.3% for romosozumab compared with teriparatide (7%) and alendronate (4%). When the drug is discontinued, there is a rapid decline in BMD.

Another possible pathway for osteoporosis treatment focuses on Cathepsin K, which is the main protease involved in osteoclast degradation of bone matrix. Odanacatib is a selective inhibitor of Cathepsin K, which inhibits bone resorption and significantly increases BMD, thereby decreasing incident fractures.[69] Recent studies showed that treatment with odanacatib for up to 8 years resulted in gains in BMD and is well tolerated.

SUMMARY

Current approaches to the treatment of osteoporosis are based on BMD and fracture risk assessment. Bisphosphonates are typically the first-line agents. A treatment failure is considered when significant loss in BMD is seen or the patient sustains a fracture despite ongoing treatment. A drug holiday is considered after 3 to 5 years of bisphosphonate treatment. Goal-directed treatment has been recently proposed based on BMD or fracture risk assessment using the FRAX tool in order to aim for a reduction of fracture risk[70] This new paradigm may help physicians to manage osteoporosis with the least potential for adverse effects.

REFERENCES

1. Center J, Nguyen TV, Schneider D, et al. Mortality after all major types of osteoporotic fracture in men and women: an observational study. Lancet 1999;353: 878–82.
2. Silverman S, Christiansen C. Individualizing osteoporosis therapy. Osteoporos Int 2012;23:797–809.
3. Lin JT, Lane JM. Rehabilitation of the older adult with an osteoporosis-related fracture. Clin Geriatr Med 2006;22:435–47.
4. Rapp K, Rothenbacher D, Magaziner J, et al. Risk of nursing home admission after femoral fracture compared with stroke, myocardial infarction, and pneumonia. J Am Med Dir Assoc 2015;16(8):715.e7-12.
5. Solomon DH, Johnston SS, Boytsov NN, et al. Osteoporosis medication use after hip fracture in U.S. Patients between 2002 and 2011. J Bone Miner Res 2014; 29(9):1929–37.
6. Kanis JA, McCloskey EV, Johansson E, et al. A reference standard for the description of osteoporosis. Bone 2008;42:467–75.
7. Khosla S. Minireview: the OPG/RANKL/RANK system. Endocrinology 2001; 142(12):5050–5.
8. Khosla S, Melton LJ 3rd, Riggs BL, et al. The unitary model for estrogen deficiency and the pathogenesis of osteoporosis: is a revision needed? J Bone Miner Res 2010;26(3):441–51.
9. Lim SY, Bolster MB. Current approaches to osteoporosis treatment. Curr Opin Rheumatol 2015;27(3):216–24.
10. Duque G, Troen BR. Understanding the mechanisms of senile osteoporosis: new facts for a major geriatric syndrome. J Am Geriatr Soc 2008;56(5):935–41.
11. Kiebzak GM, Beinart GA, Perser K, et al. Undertreatment of osteoporosis in men with hip fractures. Arch Intern Med 2002;162:2217–22.
12. Feldstein AC, Nichols G, Orwoll E, et al. The near absence of osteoporosis treatment in older men with fractures. Osteoporos Int 2005;16:953–62.
13. Abbasi AA, Rudman D, Wilson CR, et al. Observations on nursing home patient with history of hip fracture. Am J Med Sci 1995;310:229–34.
14. Ebeling PR. Osteoporosis in men. N Engl J Med 2008;358(14):1474–82.
15. Behre H, Kliesch S, Leifke E, et al. Long-term effect of testosterone therapy on bone mineral density in hypogonadal men. J Clin Endocrinol Metab 1997;82(8): 2386–90.
16. Cosman F, de Beur SJ, LeBoff MS, et al. Clinician's guide to prevention and treatment of osteoporosis. Osteoporos Int 2014;25:2359–81.
17. U.S. Preventive Services Task Force. Screening for osteoporosis: U.S. Preventive Services Task Force recommendation statement. Ann Intern Med 2011;154(5): 356–64.
18. N.O.F.a.I.S.f.C. Recommendations to DXA Manufacturers for FRAX® Implementation. Available at: www.nof.org/files/nof/public/content/resource/862/files/392. pdf. Accessed March 1, 2016.

19. Watts NB, Adler RA, Bilezikian JP, et al. Osteoporosis in men: an Endocrine Society clinical practice guideline. J Clin Endocrinol Metab 2012;97(6):1802–22.
20. Giangregorio LM, Leslie WD, Lix LM, et al. FRAX underestimates fracture risk in patients with diabetes. J Bone Miner Res 2011;27(2):301–8.
21. Black DM, Bauer DC, Schwartz AV, et al. Continuing bisphosphonate treatment for osteoporosis–for whom and for how long? N Engl J Med 2012;366(22):2051–3.
22. Hinton PS, Nigh P, Thyfault J, et al. Effectiveness of resistance training or jumping-exercise to increase bone mineral density in men with low bone mass: a 12-month randomized, clinical trial. Bone 2015;79:203–12.
23. Black DM, Rosen CJ. Postmenopausal osteoporosis. N Engl J Med 2016;374(3): 254–62.
24. Ebeling P, Wark JD, Stella J, et al. Effects of calcitriol or calcium on bone mineral density, bone turnover, and fractures in men with primary osteoporosis: a two-year randomized, double blind, double placebo study. J Clin Endocrinol Metab 2001;86(9):4098–103.
25. Murad MH, Drake MT, Mullan RJ, et al. Comparative effectiveness of drug treatments to prevent fragility fractures: a systemic review and network meta-analysis. J Clin Endocrinol Metab 2012;97:1871–80.
26. Jackson RD, LaCroix AZ, Gass M, et al. Calcium plus vitamin D supplementation and the risk of fractures. N Engl J Med 2006;354:669–83.
27. Amory JK, Watts NB, Easley KA, et al. Exogenous testosterone or testosterone with finasteride increases bone mineral density in older men with low serum testosterone. J Clin Endocrinol Metab 2004;89(2):503–10.
28. Ettinger B, Black DM, Mitlak B, et al. Reduction of vertebral fracture risk in postmenopausal women with osteoporosis treated with raloxifene: results from a 3-year randomized clinical trial. JAMA 1999;282(7):637–45.
29. Cummings SR, Tice JA, Bauer S, et al. Prevention of breast cancer in postmenopausal women: approaches to estimating and reducing risk. J Natl Cancer Inst 2009;101:384–98.
30. Black DM, Cummings SR, Karpf DB, et al. Randomized trial of effect of alendronate on risk of fracture in women with existing vertebral fractures. Lancet 1996; 348:1535–41.
31. Cummings SR, Black DM, Thompson DE, et al. Effect of alendronate on risk of fracture in women with low bone density but without vertebral fractures: results from the Fracture Intervention Trial. JAMA 1998;280:2077–82.
32. Harris ST, Watts NB, Genant HK, et al. Effects of risedronate treatment on vertebral and nonvertebral fractures in women with postmenopausal osteoporosis: a randomized controlled trial. JAMA 1999;282:1344–52.
33. Reginster J, Minne HW, Sorensen OH, et al. Randomized trial of the effects of risedronate on vertebral fractures in women with established postmenopausal osteoporosis. Osteoporos Int 2000;11:83–91.
34. McClung MR, Geusens P, Miller PD, et al. Effect of risedronate on the risk of hip fracture in elderly women. N Engl J Med 2001;344:333–40.
35. Chestnut CH, Skag A, Christiansen C, et al. Effects of oral ibandronate administered daily or intermittently on fracture risk in postmenopausal osteoporosis. J Bone Miner Res 2004;19:1241–9.
36. Reginster JY, Adami S, Lakatos P, et al. Efficacy and tolerability of once-monthly oral ibandronate in postmenopausal osteoporosis: 2 year results from the MOBILE study. Ann Rheum Dis 2006;65(5):654.

37. Eisman JA, Civitelli R, Adami S, et al. Efficacy and tolerability of intravenous ibandronate injections in postmenopausal osteoporosis: 2-year results from the DIVA study. J Rheumatol 2008;35:488–97.
38. Black DM, Delmas PD, Eastell R, et al. Once-yearly zoledronic acid for treatment of postmenopausal osteoporosis. N Engl J Med 2007;356(18):1809–22.
39. Reid IR, Gamble GD, Mesenbrink P, et al. Characterization of and risk factors for the acute-phase response after zolendronic acid. J Clin Endocrinol Metab 2010; 95:4380–7.
40. Minyan L, Guo L, Yu P, et al. Efficacy of zoledronic acid in treatment of osteoporosis in men and women—a meta-analysis. Int J Clin Exp Med 2015;8(3):3855–61.
41. Reginster JY, Neuprez A, Dardenne N, et al. Efficacy and safety of currently marketed antiosteoporosis medications. Best Pract Res Clin Endocrinol 2014; 28(809):809–34.
42. Papapoulos S, Lippuner K, Roux C, et al. The effect of 8 or 5 years of denosumab treatment in postmenopausal women with osteoporosis: results from the FREEDOM Extension study. Osteoporos Int 2015;26(12):2773.
43. Miller PD, Bolognese MA, Lewiecki M, et al. Effect of Denosumab on bone density and turnover in postmenopausal women with low bone mass after long-term continued, discontinued, and restarting of therapy: a randomized blinded phase 2 clinical trial. Bone 2008;43(2):222–9.
44. Watts NB, Roux C, Modlin JF, et al. Infections in postmenopausal women with osteoporosis treated with denosumab or placebo: coincidence or casual association? Osteoporos Int 2012;23:327–37.
45. Silva BC, Costa AG, Cusano NE, et al. Catabolic and anabolic actions of parathyroid hormone on the skeleton. J Endocrinol Invest 2011;34:801–10.
46. Neer RM, Arnaud CD, Zanchetta JR, et al. Effect of parathyroid hormone (1-34) on fractures and bone mineral density in postmenopausal women with osteoporosis. N Engl J Med 2001;344:1434–41.
47. Black DM, Bilezikian JP, Ensrud KE, et al. One year of alendronate after one year of parathyroid hormone (1-84) for osteoporosis. N Engl J Med 2005;353:555–65.
48. Leder BZ, Tsai JN, Uihlein A, et al. Denosumab and teriparatide transitions in postmenopausal osteoporosis (the DATA-Switch study): extension of a randomised controlled trial. Lancet 2015;386(9999):1147.
49. Suresh E, Pazianas M, Abrahamsen B, et al. Safety issues with biphosphonate therapy for osteoporosis. Rheumatology 2014;53:19–31.
50. Khan AA, Morrison A, Hanley DA, et al. Diagnosis and management of osteonecrosis of the jaw: a systematic review and international consensus. J Bone Miner Res 2015;30:3–23.
51. Schilcher J, Koeppen V, Aspenberg P, et al. Risk of atypical femoral fracture during and after bisphosphonate use. N Engl J Med 2014;371:974–6.
52. Feldstein AC, Black D, Perrin N, et al. Incidence and demography of femur fractures with and without atypical features. J Bone Miner Res 2012;27:977–86.
53. Favus MJ. Bisphosphonates for osteoporosis. N Engl J Med 2010;363(21): 2027–35.
54. Gedmintas L, Solomon DH, Kim SC, et al. Bisphosphonates and risk of subtrochanteric, femoral shaft, and atypical femur fracture: a systematic review and meta-analysis. J Bone Miner Res 2013;28:1729–37.
55. Dell RM, Adams AL, Greene DF, et al. Incidence of atypical nontraumatic diaphyseal fractures of the femur. J Bone Miner Res 2012;27(12):2544–50.
56. Im GI, Lee SH. Effect of teriparatide on healing of atypical femoral fractures: a systemic review. J Bone Miner Metab 2015;22(4):183–9.

57. Schilcher J, Michaëlsson K, Aspenberg P, et al. Bisphosphonate use and atypical fractures of the femoral shaft. N Engl J Med 2011;364(18):1728–37.
58. Black DM, Schwartz AV, Ensrud KA, et al. Effects of continuing or stopping alendronate after 5 years of treatment the fracture intervention trial long-term extension (FLEX): a randomized trial. JAMA 2006;296(24):2927–38.
59. Black DM, Reid IR, Boonen S, et al. The effect of 3 versus 6 years of zoledronic acid treatment of osteoporosis: a randomized extension to the HORIZON-Pivotal Fracture Trial (PFT). J Bone Miner Res 2012;27(2):243–54.
60. Black DM, Reid IR, Cauley JA, et al. The effect of 6 versus 9 years of zoledronic acid treatment in osteoporosis: a randomized second extension to the HORIZON-Pivotal Fracture Trial (PFT). J Bone Miner Res 2015;30(5):934–44.
61. Rodan G, Reszka A, Golub E, et al. Bone safety of long-term bisphosphonate treatment. Curr Med Res Opin 2004;20(8):1291.
62. Bauer DC, Schwartz A, Palermo L, et al. Fracture prediction after discontinuation of 4 to 5 years of alendronate therapy: the FLEX study. JAMA Intern Med 2014; 174(7):1126–34.
63. Schwartz AV, Bauer DC, Cummings SR, et al. Efficacy of continued alendronate for fractures in women with and without prevalent vertebral fracture: the FLEX trial. J Bone Miner Res 2010;25(5):976–82.
64. Cosman F, Cauley JA, Eastell R, et al. Reassessment of fracture risk in women after 3 years of treatment with zoledronic acid: when is it reasonable to discontinue treatment? J Clin Endocrinol Metab 2015;99(12):4546–54.
65. Reid IR, Black DM, Eastell R, et al. Reduction in the risk of clinical fractures after a single dose of zoledronic Acid 5 milligrams. J Clin Endocrinol Metab 2013;98(2): 557–63.
66. Leder BZ, O'Dea LS, Zanchetta JR, et al. Effects of abaloparatide, a human parathyroid hormone-related peptide analog, on bone mineral density in postmenopausal women with osteoporosis. J Clin Endocrinol Metab 2015;100(2):697–706.
67. Miller P, Leder BZ, Hattersley G, et al. LB-OR01-3 Effects of abaloparatide on vertebral and non-vertebral fracture incidence in postmenopausal women with osteoporosis: results of the phase 3 active trial. Paper presented at the Endocrine Society's 97th Annual Meeting & Expo. San Diego, CA, March 5, 2015.
68. McClung ML, Grauer A, Boonen S, et al. Romosozumab in postmenopausal women with low bone mineral density. N Engl J Med 2014;370(5):412–20.
69. Feng S, Luo Z, Liu D. Efficacy and safety of odanacatib treatment for patients with osteoporosis: a meta-analysis. J Bone Miner Metab 2015;33(4):448–54.
70. Cummings SR, Cosman F, Eastell R, et al. Goal-directed treatment of osteoporosis. J Bone Miner Res 2013;28:433–8.

Nonsurgical Management of Osteoarthritis Knee Pain in the Older Adult

Nora Taylor, MD

KEYWORDS

• Osteoarthritis • Management • Pharmacologic • Nonpharmacologic

KEY POINTS

• Knee osteoarthritis pain relief in older individuals often involves a mix of nonpharmacologic and pharmacologic therapies to achieve maximum benefit.
• Nonpharmacologic therapy in the form of exercise and weight loss, when appropriate, should be emphasized in all elderly patients with knee osteoarthritis to augment pharmacologic therapy.
• Treatment recommendations for older individuals should account for medical comorbidities, patient preference for modality of treatment, and functional status.

INTRODUCTION

The lifetime risk of symptomatic knee osteoarthritis is 44.7% and disproportionately affects elderly patients.[1] With a growing proportion of the population 65 years of age and older, it is estimated that the United States will have 83.7 million older adults by the year 2050.[2] Older adults opting for knee replacement are likely to suffer longer hospital stays and higher risks of both intensive care unit admission and postoperative complications as compared with younger patients.[3] As a result of patient preference and/or medical comorbidities, health care providers need to be prepared to care for and counsel older patients suffering from knee osteoarthritis who are opting to forego total joint replacement. A review of the most recent evidence regarding nonpharmacologic and pharmacologic management techniques for the older adult with knee osteoarthritis is covered here. Successful programs should be designed to meet the needs of the individual and may require multiple modalities to achieve pain reduction and improved function (**Fig. 1**).

Disclosure Statement: The author has nothing to disclose.
Division of Rheumatology, The George Washington University, 2300 M Street Northwest, Suite 307, Washington, DC 20037, USA
E-mail address: ntaylor@mfa.gwu.edu

Clin Geriatr Med 33 (2017) 41–51
http://dx.doi.org/10.1016/j.cger.2016.08.004
0749-0690/17/© 2016 Elsevier Inc. All rights reserved.

geriatric.theclinics.com

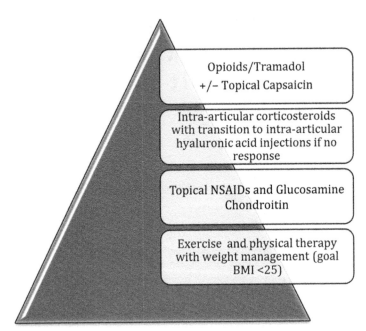

Opioids/Tramadol
+/− Topical Capsaicin

Intra-articular corticosteroids
with transition to intra-articular
hyaluronic acid injections if no
response

Topical NSAIDs and Glucosamine
Chondroitin

Exercise and physical therapy
with weight management (goal
BMI <25)

Fig. 1. Recommendations by the author for the treatment of osteoarthritis in the elderly.

NONPHARMACOLOGIC TREATMENT OPTIONS

- Nonpharmacologic management of knee osteoarthritis should focus on exercise and achieving a healthy weight.
- A 7% to 10% weight loss in obese elderly patients with symptomatic knee osteoarthritis should be the aim to achieve pain relief.
- Exercise should be tailored to the individual functional level with progressive programs favored.

WEIGHT LOSS

With the rising obesity epidemic in the United States, a large number of elderly patients with knee osteoarthritis will be clinically overweight. It is estimated that one-third of individuals over the age of 60 are obese.[4] Weight loss has been shown to decrease both pain and further cartilage loss. In a study by Gersing and colleagues,[5] a weight loss of greater than 10% over a 48-month time period slowed continued knee cartilage degeneration as measured by T2 images on MRI. Decreased progression of cartilage degeneration was best seen in the medial tibia. Among participants in the study with a greater than 10% weight loss, a statistically significant improvement in pain was measured by the Western Ontario and McMaster Universities Osteoarthritis Index (WOMAC) scales for pain and disability. The average age in each group studied was 62 (the study included patients between ages 45 and 79), and improvement in symptoms was not age dependent. In a study of 192 individuals with an average age of 62.5 years and an average body mass index (BMI) of 37 mg/m^2, a structured weight loss program over 16 weeks determined that 64% of patients had significant pain reduction as measured by the Outcome Measures in Rheumatology (OMERACT)–Osteoarthritis Research Society International (OARSI) Responder Criterion.[6] Clinical improvement related to weight loss was not affected by baseline structural damage, quadriceps strength, or abnormalities in the mechanical axis.

Although weight loss is a frequent recommendation in guidelines for treatment of osteoarthritis, the optimal amount of weight loss to target remains undetermined.[7,8] In an attempt to answer the question, an Australian study involving 1383 individuals with an average age of 64 years and a mean BMI of 34.4 found that a 7.7% weight loss was required to achieve significant pain reduction based on the Knee Injury and Osteoarthritis Outcome Score.[7] The unique aspect of the study was the search for a specific dose response to help guide clinicians in their discussions with patients. A study in *Obesity* evaluated a weight loss and exercise intervention aimed at achieving a 10% reduction in BMI in adults 60 years or older with a BMI $\geq$ 30. This study noted improved pain relief by WOMAC scoring and significantly improved 6-minute walk test and stair climb with an average 8.7% weight loss.[8] Weight loss in this study occurred over a 6-month time period. When counseling patients on a goal for weight reduction, a 7% to 10% weight loss appears to be sufficient to obtain relief from knee pain and improve function.

EXERCISE

Muscle mass and strength are lost in the natural aging process with a decline in strength appreciable even when muscle mass is maintained.[9] Prevention of obesity and maintaining lean body mass are likely central to ameliorating aging-related musculoskeletal changes.[10] Strength training is one mechanism to achieve this end. Exercise is included in the American College of Rheumatology (ACR), the European League Against Rheumatism (EULAR), and the OARSI recommendations for knee osteoarthritis management.[11–13] EULAR recommendations specify isometric exercise for both legs (to include the quadriceps and proximal hip girdle regions, irrespective of whether one or both knees are involved). Aerobic activity, stretching, and exercise instruction are also recommended.[13] EULAR recommendations favor programs that are "mixed" (involving both aerobic and strength training), that encourage integration of exercise into daily life, and that are progressive in nature.

Providers do not often specify the number of supervised sessions for patients undergoing therapy for knee osteoarthritis, but data from a Cochrane meta-analysis suggest that 12 or more sessions will have the best impact on pain reduction.[14] A Cochrane systematic review indicates that patients undergoing land-based exercise therapy will continue to benefit for 2 to 6 months after therapy intervention.[15] Despite these benefits, economic or transportation issues may limit the ability of patients to participate in physical therapy programs. In this case, providers may direct patients to online resources (eg, http://orthoinfo.org/PDFs/Rehab_Knee_6.pdf), which provide patients with home exercises that they can use routinely. Care should be taken to emphasize home safety when following self-management exercise programs so as to avoid falls and injury.

Age and functional limitation should not prevent physicians from considering a trial of physical therapy for knee osteoarthritis. To date, and despite common practice, the available data do not suggest that patients will have a greater benefit from physical therapy if they are provided with an intra-articular glucocorticoid injection before therapy.[16]

Pharmacologic Intervention: Key Points

- Topical therapies are preferred over oral therapies for osteoarthritis pain relief in the elderly to avoid medication interactions and side effects.

- Topical nonsteroidal anti-inflammatory medications (NSAIDs) and pharmaceutical grade glucosamine and chondroitin provide modest pain relief for individuals with symptomatic knee osteoarthritis along with a favorable side-effect profile.
- Intra-articular corticosteroids can provide limited duration pain improvement.
- Intra-articular hyaluronic acid injections may provide a longer duration of pain relief but are less efficacious in short-term pain relief as compared with intra-articular corticosteroids. The optimal preparation of injectable hyaluronic acid to achieve pain relief remains unclear.
- Opioids and mixed mechanism μ-receptor agonists should be reserved for cases of knee osteoarthritis that have failed standard interventions.

TOPICAL THERAPIES
Topical Nonsteroidal Anti-inflammatory Agents

Topical preparations of NSAIDs for the treatment of osteoarthritis range from over-the-counter pain balms to prescription medications. In the United States, topical diclofenac is available in a gel, solution, and patch.[17] The goal of topical preparations of NSAIDs is to achieve local anti-inflammatory effect with minimal systemic absorption. Efficacy and safety of topical NSAIDs in the treatment of osteoarthritis, collectively in trials, were evaluated in a recent review. Equal efficacy of topical NSAIDs as compared with oral NSAIDs in the treatment of knee osteoarthritis was found at 1 year.[18] The oral group experienced more respiratory adverse events and a greater increase in serum creatinine. Change of therapy in the oral NSAID group due to negative side effects was more common than in the topical NSAID group. No major adverse events, defined as death or hospitalization, were noted between the oral and topical NSAID groups. The overall low risk of adverse effects from oral NSAIDs in the trial was attributed to the strict exclusion criteria for the study. Therefore, it remains difficult to determine the relevance of these findings to an elderly population. The ACR specifically addressed adults over the age of 75 in their pharmacologic recommendations for the treatment of knee osteoarthritis by strongly recommending topical NSAID preparations over oral NSAIDs given the risk factors for oral NSAID use for adults in this age category.[12]

Although warnings regarding gastrointestinal, cardiac, and renal adverse effects are listed on package inserts for topical NSAID preparations, these side effects are only rarely reported in follow-up studies. In a report using pooled data from 3 studies of topical diclofenac for treating knee osteoarthritis, the risk of gastrointestinal events was equivalent when comparing the topical NSAID with placebo intervention groups for both patients aged 25 to 64 and those older than 65.[19] However, a significant improvement in the WOMAC pain scale for knee osteoarthritis was not observed until after week 12 in patients over the age of 65, perhaps related to more severe knee osteoarthritis in this group.

Given the safety profile of topical NSAIDs compared with oral NSAIDs in the elderly population, topical NSAIDs are an excellent initial intervention for the pharmacologic treatment of knee osteoarthritis. Because patients using the topical NSAIDs (as opposed to oral NSAIDs) report a higher level of pain at the 3-month assessment time, this may indicate that in order to achieve similar long-term effects as with oral NSAIDs, greater patience with the continued use of topical NSAIDS may be required. Topical NSAIDs are directly addressed in the OARSI guidelines for patients with isolated knee osteoarthritis and comorbidities.[13] The committee that generated these guidelines considered the quality of evidence for the endorsed use of topical NSAIDs to be "good."

Capsaicin

Capsaicin, found in the root of hot peppers, is used in topical preparations for the relief of osteoarthritis pain and is available both over the counter and by prescription. Topical capsaicin acts through depletion of type-C nociceptive nerve fibers, thereby impairing neuronal release of substance P, and ultimately modulating the local sensory response. Pain signals are dampened with recurrent capsaicin application. For knee osteoarthritis, topical capsaicin is applied in a thin layer 4 times daily in order to achieve pain relief. Local skin irritation occurs commonly, and care must be taken so as not to accidentally touch or splatter mucous membranes or the eyes.

In a review of randomized controlled trials of topical capsaicin (of which 3 of the 5 reviews specified knee osteoarthritis), Laslett and Jones[20] noted only a moderate change in the visual analogue scale (VAS) pain scale over a 4-week time period. No systemic toxicity was noted, but topical irritation was recorded in 35% to 100% of participants. The 2013 OARSI guidelines recommend the use of topical capsaicin in knee osteoarthritis patients without comorbidities but made no assertion about benefit in patients possessing comorbidities.[13] In contrast, the 2012 ACR guidelines did not recommend the use of topical capsaicin given the lack of high-quality evidence supporting its use.[12] In a 2013 *Cochrane Review* of topical herbal therapies for osteoarthritis, capsaicin (Capsicum) gel was not noted to be more effective than placebo.[21] With a high likelihood of skin irritation, and with the requirement for frequent application, along with insufficient evidence of efficacy, the pragmatic use of capsaicin treatment might be reserved for the situation of an older patient seeking to forestall a trial of opioid therapy.

Intra-articular Corticosteroid Injections

Intra-articular corticosteroid injections are used by physicians frequently in the care of osteoarthritis knee pain and are performed by primary care physicians, geriatricians, orthopedists, and rheumatologists. Intra-articular corticosteroid injections are an in-office procedure with significant appeal for both physician and patient given the excellent safety profile and lack of systemic side effects.[22] However, pain relief may be variable in degree and modest in duration. The EULAR, OARSI, and ACR guidelines all include recommendations for the use of intra-articular corticosteroids for the treatment of knee osteoarthritis pain. Contraindications to injection include infection at the injection site, sepsis, or a preexisting knee replacement.

Based on a *Cochrane Review* of intra-articular corticosteroids for knee osteoarthritis that pooled 27 studies with 1767 total participants, intra-articular glucocorticoids improved pain relief by a difference of 1.0 cm on a 10-cm VAS as compared with sham injections.[23] The therapeutic effect of injections does not have a prolonged duration. A small to moderate benefit compared with placebo was observed 4 to 6 weeks after injection; a small effect was observed at 13 weeks, and no difference was noted at 26 weeks. Patients may require repeat injections for pain relief, although the safe interval between injections and optimal preparation of steroid has yet to be established.[24] There are no predictors of response to intra-articular steroid injections based on available data to date, making it difficult to counsel patients regarding the likelihood that they will respond to an injection. Data for the use of intra-articular corticosteroids are stronger than that of intra-articular hyaluronic acid (IA-HA) injections with regards to short-term pain relief; however, with time, IA-HA appears more efficacious for pain relief.[25] Most studies evaluate patients in the sixth decade. No study specifically addresses the benefit of intra-articular steroids in the very elderly.

Performing intra-articular glucocorticoid injections in older adults may require special advance preparation and positional aides in order to work around patient limitations. Patients who are unable to move to the examination table or are unable to extend their knee may have injections via an anterior infrapatellar lateral or medial approach. Utilization of the infrapatellar approach with the knee flexed to 90° and aiming toward the midline is a well-tolerated and popular technique among rheumatologists. The anterior-lateral infrapatellar approach may have improved accuracy data as compared with the anterior-infrapatellar medial approach in this situation.[26]

If knee anatomy is distorted by advanced osteoarthritis or body habitus, image-guided injection should be considered. One of every 5 nonvisualized knee injections does not enter the intra-articular space (a number that may be higher for inexperienced physicians or in cases of patients with challenging anatomy). Bedside ultrasound-guided injection is an appealing option. Ultrasound-guided injections provide better short-term outcomes and less injection site complications as compared with blinded injections. However, long-term outcomes appear to be similar between image-guided and palpation-guided injections.[27]

Intra-articular Hyaluronic Acid Injections

Conflicting data exist for the use of IA-HA injections for the treatment of knee osteoarthritis. First approved in 1997, viscosupplementation was thought to improve shock absorption and provide improved lubrication and pain relief in the knee. Different preparations of IA-HAs are marketed, and the frequency of injection ranges from single-dose injection (eg, Synvisc-One) to multidose injections given as a series once weekly over several weeks (eg, Euflexxa). Guidelines from the ACR make no specific recommendations regarding the use of IA-HA injections beyond noting that their use may be appropriate for individuals 75 years of age and older and who cannot take oral NSAIDs.[12] OARSI guidelines report "uncertain" benefit in the use of IA-HA for knee osteoarthritis.[13] More recently, the European Society for Clinical and Economic Aspects of Osteoporosis and Osteoarthritis (ESCEO) published recommendations for the use of IA-HA injections in patients who have an inadequate response to NSAID use.[28] Given the risks to older patients from chronic NSAID use, IA-HA injections may be more appropriate. A multi-center trial has demonstrated equal short-term efficacy between these 2 therapies.[29]

Meta-analyses of the use of IA-HA injections for osteoarthritis pain suffer from confounding due to heterogeneity in the preparations and also due to lack of appropriately designed double-blind placebo controlled trials. Pain relief is also variable among the different studies of IA-HA injections. Intra-articular corticosteroids appear to have better short-term effect on pain control. Whereas, IA-HA injections may have improved pain relief at the 8-week mark.[27] Potential residual effect is up to 24 weeks in some studies. The reported effect size in a 2011 meta-analysis of IA-HA injections was 0.46 (>0.20 is considered clinically relevant), which was greater than that for acetaminophen and NSAIDs.[30] The optimal preparation of IA-HA agent is not known, but there is evidence that patients may derive greater benefit from higher-molecular-weight IA-HAs.[31] Berenbaum and colleagues[32] in a 2012 study found a higher proportion of OMERACT-OARSI responders with high-molecular-weight IA-HA (73%) versus the intermediate-molecular-weight IA-HA preparations (58%) at the 6-month mark. Despite these findings, there remains insufficient evidence to support the use of one IA-HA preparation over another.

A systematic review of the effectiveness of IA-HA injections on physical functioning for those patients with severe degenerative osteoarthritis with an average age of 65 or older revealed a small but statistically significant improvement with few serious adverse effects.[33] However, when only double-blinded, sham-controlled trials are considered, no therapeutic difference is observed between IA-HA injections and placebo. Therefore, although the benefit to older adults appears less than certain, IA-HA remains a viable option owing in large part to its relative safety profile.[34]

ORAL THERAPIES
Nonsteroidal Anti-inflammatory Drugs

NSAIDs have strong data to support their use for pain relief in osteoarthritis. Unfortunately, the deleterious effects to kidneys, as well as to the cardiovascular and gastrointestinal systems, make them a riskier choice in older adults.[35,36] Cyclooxygenase-2 inhibitors (COX-2), such as Celecoxib, possess reduced gastrointestinal toxicity but remain a concern with regards to cardiovascular risk.[37] Given the risk profile of both NSAIDs and COX-2 inhibitors, the author favors sporadic use with careful monitoring in otherwise healthy patients between 65 and 75 years of age and avoids their use altogether in patients 75 and older.

Acetaminophen

Acetaminophen is widely used in the management of osteoarthritis of the knee. Its use is recommended by the ACR for the management of osteoarthritis, and it is considered "appropriate" for use in patients without relevant comorbidities (OARSI treatment guidelines).[12,13] Although acetaminophen is relatively safe for younger individuals without comorbidities, it may confer a greater risk in frail older adults and also may not provide as substantial pain relief as once hoped.[35] In a *Cochrane Review* in 2006 evaluating the efficacy of acetaminophen in treating hip and knee osteoarthritis, the number needed to treat with acetaminophen to achieve a 5% pain reduction ranged from 4 to 16 individuals.[38] In the situation of liver impairment, acetaminophen is contraindicated. If acetaminophen is to be used for pain control, doses up to 4 g daily (and continuously) are often required in order to achieve a modest pain relief benefit. Therefore, care must be taken to evaluate the medication list of all patients using high-dose acetaminophen in order to ensure that underappreciated ingestion of other acetaminophen-containing medications does not place individuals at increased risk for toxicity.

Glucosamine and Chondroitin

The use of glucosamine and chondroitin has undergone significant scrutiny over the past decade. The Glucosamine/chondroitin Arthritis Intervention Trial found no evidence for effective pain reduction in knee osteoarthritis; however, subgroup analysis noted a trend toward pain relief in patients with moderate to severe knee pain.[39] Previous evaluations of glucosamine sulfate have found that only the crystalline glucosamine sulfate formulations were associated with significant pain and structural benefits. Chondroitin may also provide a modest benefit with regards to pain relief. In a recent *Cochrane Review* of the effects of chondroitin on osteoarthritis pain, it was found that patients experience an average 8-point (scale 0–100) reduction in pain using chondroitin while enduring fewer side effects than placebo.[40] Although this review looked primarily at patients with knee osteoarthritis, some of the included trials examined patients with hip and hand osteoarthritis as well.

Recent guidelines for the management of symptomatic knee osteoarthritis published by the ESCEO suggest use of prescription dose (1500 mg) of patented crystalline glucosamine sulfate as a first-line therapy.[28] Use of patented crystalline glucosamine sulfate has similar efficacy to NSAIDs, and possibly better efficacy than that reported for paracetamol or acetaminophen preparations.[41] Chondroitin, either used in combination with glucosamine or alone, was also recommended as a first-line treatment. Some yet to be replicated studies report a reduction in joint space narrowing with the use of combination pharmaceutical grade glucosamine and chondroitin with fewer adverse events compared with placebo.[42,43] The safety profile of glucosamine and chondroitin makes them attractive agents in elderly patients. However, difficulty in obtaining prescription grade glucosamine and/or chondroitin may limit their use.

Tramadol and Other Opioids

Use of opioid analgesics in the treatment of knee osteoarthritis in the elderly may pose challenges owing to tolerability, increased fall risk, withdrawal, and constipation. Elderly patients may experience age-related decline in clearance of opiates from their system in addition to a risk of polypharmacy reducing efficacy or leading to adverse outcomes.[44] Geriatric Society Guidelines address these concerns in the 2009 report on pharmacologic management of persistent pain in older adults.[45] Opioid management of knee osteoarthritis pain should be considered on a trial basis initially and with strict follow-up for management and monitoring. The increase of opioid misuse and accidental deaths has led to evolving steps by the US Health and Human Services Secretary and Centers for Disease Control and Prevention to address opioid-prescribing practices with a focus on utilization of the minimally effective dose.[46,47] Specific reference is made to utilization of a multimodal approach to pain management when opioids are used.

Tramadol and tapentadol, analgesics with activity on the μ-opiod receptor as well as norepinephrine and serotonin reuptake inhibition, are generally reserved for refractory knee pain in patients who have failed other pain management modalities. Tramadol and tapentadol should be considered when all alternate options have been exhausted and the patient remains hampered by daily knee pain.[48] Short- and long-acting preparations are available to allow practitioners to develop optimized dosing schedules for their patients. Data suggest that the benefit of opioids in the treatment of osteoarthritis pain is similar to that of NSAIDs. The effect of mixed mechanism μ-opiod agonists and opiates in the treatment of knee osteoarthritis is equivalent as per the OARSI.[13] For this reason, many practitioners favor the use of tramadol when opioid-agonist therapy is deemed necessary.

If opioids are not effective in achieving a substantial decrease in osteoarthritis knee pain, then these agents should be discontinued as soon as possible to minimize tolerance, dependence, and potential for adverse side effects. In a 2014 *Cochrane Review*, oral and transdermal opioids for the treatment of knee and hip osteoarthritis improved both function and pain scores. An average 0.7-mm improvement in pain on a 10-mm VAS was noted with the use of opioids compared with placebo.[49] This modest benefit in pain relief was associated with a 22% opioid side-effect rate. A recent review and comparison of 27 randomized controlled trials comparing NSAIDs, tramadol, and opioids revealed similar rates of pain relief among the medications, suggesting that providers should choose the safest option for their particular patient when discussing oral therapies.[50]

SUMMARY

The nonsurgical care of the elderly patient with symptomatic knee osteoarthritis should consist of combination treatment with nonpharmacologic and pharmacologic modalities. Goals should be aimed at pain reduction and improved function while minimizing potential negative side effects, in particular those associated with long-term oral opioid use. Progressive exercise programs and weight loss remain pillars of non-pharmacologic therapy. Topical NSAIDs and pharmaceutical grade glucosamine and/or chondroitin can provide modest pain relief with minimal potential adverse effects. Intra-articular injections of corticosteroids and IA-HA injections are generally safe and well tolerated by elderly patients and should be used to augment pain relief.

REFERENCES

1. Murphy L, Schwartz TA, Helmick CG, et al. Lifetime risk of symptomatic knee osteoarthritis. Arthritis Rheum 2008;59(9):1207–13.
2. Ortman JV, V. 2014. Available at: https://www.census.gov/prod/2014pubs/p25-1140.pdf.
3. Fang M, Noiseux N, Linson E, et al. The effect of advancing age on total joint replacement outcomes. Geriatr Orthop Surg Rehabil 2015;6(3):173–9.
4. Porter Starr KN, Bales CW. Excessive body weight in older adults. Clin Geriatr Med 2015;31(3):311–26.
5. Gersing AS, Solka M, Joseph GB, et al. Progression of cartilage degeneration and clinical symptoms in obese and overweight individuals is dependent on the amount of weight loss: 48-month data from the Osteoarthritis Initiative. Osteoarthritis Cartilage 2016;24(7):1126–34.
6. Gudbergsen H, Boesen M, Lohmander LS, et al. Weight loss is effective for symptomatic relief in obese subjects with knee osteoarthritis independently of joint damage severity assessed by high-field MRI and radiography. Osteoarthritis Cartilage 2012;20(6):495–502.
7. Atukorala I, Makovey J, Lawler L, et al. Is there a dose response relationship between weight loss and symptom improvement in persons with knee osteoarthritis? Arthritis Care Res (Hoboken) 2016;68(8):1106–14.
8. Miller GD, Nicklas BJ, Davis C, et al. Intensive weight loss program improves physical function in older obese adults with knee osteoarthritis. Obesity (Silver Spring) 2006;14(7):1219–30.
9. Goodpaster BH, Park SW, Harris TB, et al. The loss of skeletal muscle strength, mass, and quality in older adults: the health, aging and body composition study. J Gerontol A Biol Sci Med Sci 2006;61(10):1059–64.
10. Fielding RA. The role of progressive resistance training and nutrition in the preservation of lean body mass in the elderly. J Am Coll Nutr 1995;14(6):587–94.
11. Fernandes L, Hagen KB, Bijlsma JW, et al. EULAR recommendations for the non-pharmacological core management of hip and knee osteoarthritis. Ann Rheum Dis 2013;72(7):1125–35.
12. Hochberg MC, Altman RD, April KT, et al. American College of Rheumatology 2012 recommendations for the use of nonpharmacologic and pharmacologic therapies in osteoarthritis of the hand, hip, and knee. Arthritis Care Res (Hoboken) 2012;64(4):465–74.
13. McAlindon TE, Bannuru RR, Sullivan MC, et al. OARSI guidelines for the non-surgical management of knee osteoarthritis. Osteoarthritis Cartilage 2014;22(3):363–88.
14. Fransen M, McConnell S. Land-based exercise for osteoarthritis of the knee: a metaanalysis of randomized controlled trials. J Rheumatol 2009;36(6):1109–17.
15. Fransen M, McConnell S, Harmer AR, et al. Exercise for osteoarthritis of the knee: a Cochrane systematic review. Br J Sports Med 2015;49(24):1554–7.

16. Henriksen M, Christensen R, Klokker L, et al. Evaluation of the benefit of cortico-steroid injection before exercise therapy in patients with osteoarthritis of the knee: a randomized clinical trial. JAMA Intern Med 2015;175(6):923–30.

17. McPherson ML, Cimino NM. Topical NSAID formulations. Pain Med 2013; 14(Suppl 1):S35–9.

18. Underwood M, Ashby D, Cross P, et al. Advice to use topical or oral ibuprofen for chronic knee pain in older people: randomised controlled trial and patient prefer-ence study. BMJ 2008;336(7636):138–42.

19. Baraf HS, Gloth FM, Barthel HR, et al. Safety and efficacy of topical diclofenac sodium gel for knee osteoarthritis in elderly and younger patients: pooled data from three randomized, double-blind, parallel-group, placebo-controlled, multi-centre trials. Drugs Aging 2011;28(1):27–40.

20. Laslett LL, Jones G. Capsaicin for osteoarthritis pain. Prog Drug Res 2014;68: 277–91.

21. Cameron M, Chrubasik S. Topical herbal therapies for treating osteoarthritis. Co-chrane Database Syst Rev 2013;(5):CD010538.

22. Cardone DA, Tallia AF. Joint and soft tissue injection. Am Fam Physician 2002; 66(2):283–8.

23. Juni P, Hari R, Rutjes AW, et al. Intra-articular corticosteroid for knee osteoarthritis. Cochrane Database Syst Rev 2015;(10):CD005328.

24. Douglas RJ. Corticosteroid injection into the osteoarthritic knee: drug selection, dose, and injection frequency. Int J Clin Pract 2012;66(7):699–704.

25. Bannuru RR, Natov NS, Obadan IE, et al. Therapeutic trajectory of hyaluronic acid versus corticosteroids in the treatment of knee osteoarthritis: a systematic review and meta-analysis. Arthritis Rheum 2009;61(12):1704–11.

26. Douglas RJ. Aspiration and injection of the knee joint: approach portal. Knee Surg Relat Res 2014;26(1):1–6.

27. Maricar N, Parkes MJ, Callaghan MJ, et al. Where and how to inject the knee–a systematic review. Semin Arthritis Rheum 2013;43(2):195–203.

28. Bruyere O, Cooper C, Pelletier JP, et al. A consensus statement on the European Society for Clinical and Economic Aspects of Osteoporosis and Osteoarthritis (ESCEO) algorithm for the management of knee osteoarthritis-From evidence-based medicine to the real-life setting. Semin Arthritis Rheum 2016;45(4 Suppl):S3–s11.

29. Ishijima M, Nakamura T, Shimizu K, et al. Intra-articular hyaluronic acid injection versus oral non-steroidal anti-inflammatory drug for the treatment of knee osteo-arthritis: a multi-center, randomized, open-label, non-inferiority trial. Arthritis Res Ther 2014;16(1):R18.

30. Bannuru RR, Natov NS, Dasi UR, et al. Therapeutic trajectory following intra-articular hyaluronic acid injection in knee osteoarthritis–meta-analysis. Osteoar-thritis Cartilage 2011;19(6):611–9.

31. Berenbaum F, Grifka J, Cazzaniga S, et al. A randomised, double-blind, controlled trial comparing two intra-articular hyaluronic acid preparations differing by their molecular weight in symptomatic knee osteoarthritis. Ann Rheum Dis 2012;71(9):1454–60.

32. Kotevoglu N, Iyibozkurt PC, Hiz O, et al. A prospective randomised controlled clinical trial comparing the efficacy of different molecular weight hyaluronan solu-tions in the treatment of knee osteoarthritis. Rheumatol Int 2006;26(4):325–30.

33. Newberry SJ. AHRQ technology assessments, in systematic review for effective-ness of hyaluronic acid in the treatment of severe degenerative joint disease

(DJD) of the knee. Rockville (MD): Agency for Healthcare Research and Quality (US); 2015.

34. Abate M, Pulcini D, Di Iorio A, et al. Viscosupplementation with intra-articular hyaluronic acid for treatment of osteoarthritis in the elderly. Curr Pharm Des 2010; 16(6):631–40.

35. American Geriatrics Society Panel on the Pharmacological Management of Persistent Pain in Older Persons. Pharmacological management of persistent pain in older persons. Pain Med 2009;10(6):1062–83.

36. Amer M, Bead VR, Bathon J, et al. Use of nonsteroidal anti-inflammatory drugs in patients with cardiovascular disease: a cautionary tale. Cardiol Rev 2010;18(4): 204–12.

37. Scarpignato C, Lanas A, Blandizzi C, et al. Safe prescribing of non-steroidal antiinflammatory drugs in patients with osteoarthritis–an expert consensus addressing benefits as well as gastrointestinal and cardiovascular risks. BMC Med 2015; 13:55.

38. Towheed TE, Maxwell L, Judd MG, et al. Acetaminophen for osteoarthritis. Cochrane Database Syst Rev 2006;(1):CD004257.

39. Clegg DO, Reda DJ, Harris CL, et al. Glucosamine, chondroitin sulfate, and the two in combination for painful knee osteoarthritis. N Engl J Med 2006;354(8): 795–808.

40. Singh JA, Noorbaloochi S, MacDonald R, et al. Chondroitin for osteoarthritis. Cochrane Database Syst Rev 2015;(1):CD005614.

41. Herrero-Beaumont G, Ivorra JA, Del Carmen Trabado M, et al. Glucosamine sulfate in the treatment of knee osteoarthritis symptoms: a randomized, doubleblind, placebo-controlled study using acetaminophen as a side comparator. Arthritis Rheum 2007;56(2):555–67.

42. Hochberg M, Chevalier X, Henrotin Y, et al. Symptom and structure modification in osteoarthritis with pharmaceutical-grade chondroitin sulfate: what's the evidence? Curr Med Res Opin 2013;29(3):259–67.

43. Bruyere O, Reginster JY. Glucosamine and chondroitin sulfate as therapeutic agents for knee and hip osteoarthritis. Drugs Aging 2007;24(7):573–80.

44. O'Neil CK, Hanlon JT, Marcum ZA. Adverse effects of analgesics commonly used by older adults with osteoarthritis: focus on non-opioid and opioid analgesics. Am J Geriatr Pharmacother 2012;10(6):331–42.

45. American Geriatrics Society Panel on Pharmacological Management of Persistent Pain in Older Persons. Pharmacological management of persistent pain in older persons. J Am Geriatr Soc 2009;57(8):1331–46.

46. McCarthy M. Opioids should be last resort to treat chronic pain, says draft CDC guideline. BMJ 2015;351:h6905.

47. Dowell D, Haegerich TM, Chou R. CDC guideline for prescribing opioids for chronic pain–United States, 2016. JAMA 2016;315(15):1624–45.

48. Santos J, Alarcão J, Fareleira F, et al. Tapentadol for chronic musculoskeletal pain in adults. Cochrane Database Syst Rev 2015;(5):CD009923.

49. da Costa BR, Nüesch E, Kasteler R, et al. Oral or transdermal opioids for osteoarthritis of the knee or hip. Cochrane Database Syst Rev 2014;(9):CD003115.

50. Smith SR, Deshpande BR, Collins JE, et al. Comparative pain reduction of oral non-steroidal anti-inflammatory drugs and opioids for knee osteoarthritis: systematic analytic review. Osteoarthritis Cartilage 2016;24(6):962–72.

Regional Rheumatic Disorders and Rehabilitation in Older Adults

Ana T. Acevedo, MD*, Adrienne Jackson, PT, PhD, MPA,
Katharine E. Alter, MD

KEYWORDS

- Regional rheumatic pain syndromes • Geriatric rehabilitation
- Rehabilitation medicine

KEY POINTS

- To review key components of the rehabilitation medicine evaluation of older patients with regional rheumatic disorders.
- To understand the rationale behind rehabilitation medicine treatment interventions of older patients with regional rheumatic disorders.
- To review future research considerations of older patients with regional rheumatic disorders.

INTRODUCTION

Musculoskeletal (MSK) problems are the most frequently reported complaints among community-dwelling older adults.[1,2] In patients more than 60 years old, the prevalence of pain was more than 2 times that reported for patients less than 60 years old.[3,4] In developed countries, the fastest growing portion of the population are individuals who are older than 75 years of age.[4,5] The impact of the aging process on skeletal muscles and joints can have a profound effect on the functional ability of individuals with and without disabilities.[6] Despite its universal occurrence, the mechanisms of aging are not fully understood.[7,8] Structural and mechanical changes of aging occur in skeletal muscle and the articular cartilage and result in biomechanical changes that may affect mobility, self-care skills, and activities of daily living. This article reviews the rehabilitation medicine approach to the evaluation of older adults with regional rheumatic disorders and the approach to clinical intervention.

Disclosure: The authors have nothing to disclose.
Rehabilitation Medicine Department, National Institutes of Health Clinical Center, 10 Center Drive, Building 10, CRC, Room 1-1469, Bethesda, MD 20892-1604, USA
* Corresponding author.
E-mail address: ana.acevedo@nih.gov

WHAT IS A REGIONAL RHEUMATIC DISORDER?

For the purposes of this article, a regional rheumatic disorders is a localized dysfunction related to nonarticular or periarticular soft tissue. The disorder may involve the bursa, muscle, fascia, ligament, tendon, cartilage, joint, bone, nerve, or overlying skin and how these tissues relate to each other.[9] Local trauma is the most common initiating event for regional rheumatic disorders. A macrotraumatic injury involves a single episode of acute tissue destruction, whereas a microtraumatic injury can result from chronic overload[10] or repetitive overuse. Intrinsic and extrinsic factors affect these injuries and predispose to inflammation, degeneration, tear, or rupture.[10] Examples of intrinsic factors include age, biomechanical malalignments, muscle imbalances, hypermobility or hypomobility, poor vascular supply,[10] lack of exercise/movement/undermobility, and comorbidities. Tendons become less flexible and elastic with aging, making them more susceptible to injuries.[11] Extrinsic factors relate to external environmental issues that may affect the individual, such as walking on uneven surfaces, lack of access to exercise opportunities, poor exercise training techniques, or exposure to extreme temperature fluctuations.

PATIENT EVALUATION CONSIDERATIONS

Given the absence of specific standardized laboratory tests, markers, or imaging tests for regional rheumatic disorders, a comprehensive medical history and physical examination are essential. The initial medical history should differentiate whether the complaint is articular or nonarticular, inflammatory or noninflammatory, acute or chronic, and localized or widespread.[9]

Pain is often the primary symptom in patients with MSK complaints. A pain history should include pain onset, location, duration, type of pain, and associated factors that may aggravate, exacerbate, or decrease pain. Clinicians should query patients for a history of recent or remote trauma. Associated symptoms, such as weakness, edema, effusion, redness, warmth, fevers, and chills, are important in the differential diagnosis. A comprehensive functional history is critical for identifying activities that may or may not be limited to symptoms related to regional rheumatic disorders.

REHABILITATION MEDICINE HISTORY

The functional history includes an understanding of the premorbid level of functioning, which includes inquiring about transfers, mobility, walking, avocational activities, and need for mobility aids such as canes, walkers, or wheelchairs. Before the MSK complaint, was the patient independent or did the patient require some form of physical assistance from another person with or without mobility aids or adaptive equipment? The functional history of self-care and activities of daily living should include the person's skills in the areas of bathing, toileting, personal hygiene, upper and lower extremity dressing, meal preparation, home maintenance, and home and community accessibility (eg, the inability to put on deodorant or a shirt because of restricted shoulder range of motion in the case of a shoulder tendinopathy or rotator cuff tear).

In addition to gathering the traditional information, clinicians should consider some unique factors that influence the trajectory of older adults with regional rheumatic disorders from disease to disability (**Box 1**).[12–14]

An important area to address during the systems review is cognition. Because the inability to learn can negatively affect the rehabilitation program, older adults should also be screened for the following[12]:

- Communication ability (eg, ability to make needs known)
- Affect (eg, expected emotional/behavioral responses)

> **Box 1**
> **Additional factors to consider when gathering the patient's history**
>
> - Patient's/family's understanding of the disease and its implications
> - Patient's/family's goals related to rehabilitation
> - Cultural beliefs/behaviors (health beliefs)
> - Role function
> - Social support/interaction/activities
> - Exercise likes and dislikes/frequency and intensity of regular activity
> - Sexual activity
> - Recreational hobbies
> - Substance abuse
> - Family/caregiver resources
> - Methods of coping/adaptation to stress
> - Values/spirituality
> - Signs of elder abuse/mistreatment (be aware of your state's reporting requirements)

- Cognition (eg, assessment of consciousness and orientation)
- Learning style/preferences (eg, learning barriers, education needs)

PHYSICAL EXAMINATION

The physical examination should be comprehensive and include inspection; palpation; passive and active range of motions of the joints; as well as testing of muscle strength, tone, and sensation. It is imperative to evaluate for physical asymmetries, postural abnormalities, joint deformities, muscle imbalances, and limb discrepancies that may have been preexisting or result from an acute injury. In older patients, the examination should include coordination, and static and dynamic balance testing. The range-of-motion examination is particularly important, because even minor losses in range of motion can negatively affect function.[15] For example, loss of shoulder external rotation may result in the inability to wash hair. Loss of range of motion at the wrists and fingers may affect any activities requiring manual dexterity.[15] Decreased hip rotation and extension may have a negative impact on gait efficiency,[15] which may worsen in a clinical scenario of trochanteric bursitis. **Table 1** highlights unique factors that should be considered during the physical examination of older adults with regional rheumatic disorders.

SUPPLEMENTARY WORK-UP

The findings on physical examination guide additional work-up, which may include laboratory and/or imaging studies. A full discussion of either of these topics is beyond the scope of this article. However, ultrasonography (US) imaging is reviewed here, because this imaging technique is commonly used by physiatrists and has become an extension of the physical examination.[18–20]

Brightness mode (B-mode) US is widely used in clinical practice for assessment of the MSK system, including muscles, tendons, joints, ligaments, and neurovascular structures. The development of high-frequency linear US transducers has

Table 1 **Special considerations when selecting tests and measures for older adults with regional rheumatic disorders**	
ROM	Joint pain or activity tolerance may prevent traditional goniometric ROM testing. Functional ROM testing may be substituted to determine whether the older adult has the range needed to perform self-care activities[16]
Strength	Pain and joint effusion impede muscle contraction, thus limiting the examination of strength. Traditional strength testing (eg, MMT) is not appropriate in the presence of severely deformed joints. Functional strength assessments provide sufficient data to formulate treatment goals and assess outcomes[16]
Joint Mobility	With aging, connective tissue can lose elastic properties, causing increased or decreased joint mobility. Systemic conditions such as diabetes and rheumatoid arthritis are associated with impairments in joint mobility[17]
Sensory Integrity	Alterations in sensation may be evident with the presence of Raynaud disease, compression of nerves because of inflammation or joint derangement, diabetes, or normal age-related changes[16]
Cardiovascular	Heart rate, respiratory rate, blood pressure, and RPE should all be measured. Be aware of medications that may blunt heart rate or blood pressure response to exercise. Excessive increases in RPE may indicate the presence of inflammation or impairment of pulmonary and cardiac function that requires more extensive and formal evaluation[16]
Functional Assessment	A suggested first step is observational analysis of functional tasks. However, considering the lack of established reliability, observational task analysis should be used cautiously. Rather than being used independently, observational task analysis should guide the selection of additional quantitative tests and measures. The quantification of functional activity, if based on valid and reliable measures, allows clinicians to describe patient/client progression and document outcomes[17]

Abbreviations: MMT, manual muscle testing; ROM, range of motion; RPE, ratings of perceived exertion.

Data from Vlieland TPV. Multidisciplinary team care and outcomes in rheumatoid arthritis. Curr Opin Rheumatol 2004;16(2):153–6; and Federal Interagency Forum on Aging-Related Statistics. Older Americans 2012: key indicators of well-being. Washington, DC: US Government Printing Office; 2012.

revolutionized MSK imaging and produces exquisitely detailed high-resolution images and has revolutionized the imaging of many MSK structures (**Fig. 1**). US can reveal the presence of anatomic variations and disorders, including tendinopathy, tendon tears/ruptures, ligament laxity/tears, joint effusions, bursal enlargement, and muscle diseases/injury/atrophy involving MSK structures[21] (**Fig. 2**).

US imaging advantages include that it is portable, does not use ionizing radiation, and is low cost. Another advantage of US is that it can be used during dynamic assessment of patients. Examples include evaluation of impingement while moving a shoulder through its range of motion, noting abnormal ligamentous laxity when a joint is mechanically stressed, and sonopalpation of an area (using the transducer to recreate pain or observe the effects of compression). Color Doppler US is also useful for imaging the MSK system and may reveal hypervascularity or increased blood flow in areas of inflammation or neovascularization.[21,22]

US is useful for procedural guidance, including joint aspiration/injection, injections of tendons and ligaments, and/or US-guided needle tenotomy (**Fig. 3**).

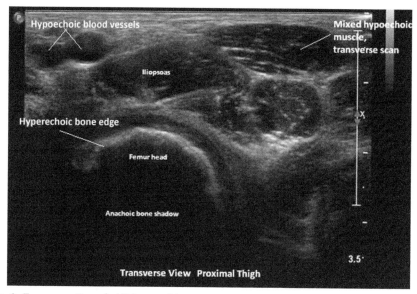

Fig. 1. Transverse B-mode US image, hip.

COMMON REGIONAL RHEUMATIC PAIN SYNDROMES

The rheumatology and physical medicine literature describing regional rheumatic syndrome is extensive.[11,23–27] The authors encourage readers to review the references listed in the References section.

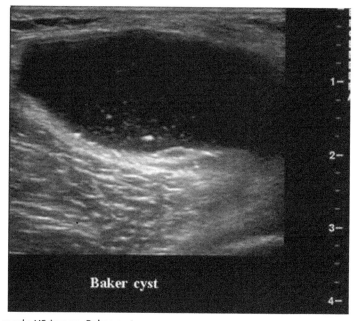

Fig. 2. B-mode US image, Baker cyst.

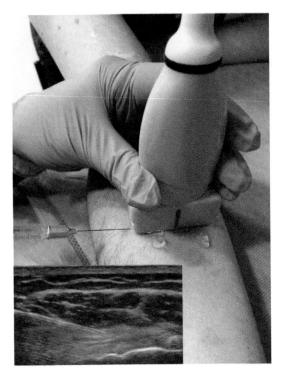

Fig. 3. In-plane needle insertion, forearm.

Bursae Disorders

Briefly, most bursae disorders are inflammatory, hence the term bursitis. The function of the bursa is to facilitate movement of tendons and muscles over bony prominences.[28] Excessive and/or repetitive motions from overuse, trauma, systemic disease, or infection may cause bursitis.[28] **Box 2** lists common types of bursitis in the clinical setting.

The medical treatment of most bursitis is straightforward and involves rest, identifying and preventing the aggravating factors, the use of nonsteroidal oral antiinflammatory agents (unless medically contraindicated), and/or the administration of a

---

Box 2
Common bursitis in the clinical setting

- Subacromial bursitis/subdeltoid bursitis of the shoulder
- Olecranon bursitis over the posterior elbow
- De Quervain tenosynovitis of the wrist
- Trochanteric bursitis of the hip
- Ischial bursitis (weaver's bottom)
- Iliopsoas bursitis
- Prepatellar bursitis of the knee (housemaid's knee)
- Anserine bursitis
- Achilles bursitis/retrocalcaneal bursitis

glucocorticoid injection. Glucocorticoid injection is usually curative and diagnostic if the diagnosis is accurate.

All injuries present with localized pain and tenderness. Clinicians should differentiate acute inflammation tendinitis) versus chronic tendon degeneration (tendinopathy) because the treatment goals and healing times differ.

Ligamentous injuries

Ligamentous injuries may result in sprains, which may be graded according to the degree of severity.
- Grade I injury: ligament is overstretched; without joint instability
- Grade II injury: ligament is partially torn; there is mild joint instability
- Grade III injury: ligament is completely torn; there is joint instability and significant bruising

Muscle or tendon injuries

Muscle or tendon injuries may result in strains, which are also graded per severity.
- Grade I injury: muscle or tendon tissue is overstretched
- Grade II injury: muscle or tendon tissue is partially torn
- Grade III injury muscle or tendon tissue is completely torn

Most strains present with swelling, bruising, pain, local warmth, and/or local nodule or point tenderness and dysfunction. Complete tears are suspected in cases of weakness, and complete disruption of movement. In cases of severe disruption and instability, a secondary nerve impingement may occur. **Box 3** lists common tendinopathies in the clinical setting.

SPECIFIC TESTS

In order to differentiate the various entities and degree of injury, clinicians may rely on specific tests. For example, the drop-arm test, in which the examiner passively abducts the patient's shoulder 90°. The patient is then asked to slowly lower the arm back to the side. A positive test result is indicated by the patient's inability to

---

Box 3
Common tendinopathies in the clinical setting

- Shoulder rotator cuff tendinopathy
- Shoulder rotator cuff tear (complete or incomplete)
- Proximal bicipital tendinitis/tendinopathy
- Adhesive capsulitis (frozen shoulder)
- Lateral elbow epicondylitis (tennis elbow)
- Medial elbow epicondylitis (golfer's elbow)
- Triceps tendon rupture
- Tenosynovitis of the wrist
- Popliteal tendinitis of the knee/tendinopathy
- Patellar tendinitis/tendinopathy
- Achilles tendinitis/tendinopathy
- Posterior tibialis tendon tendinitis or rupture

voluntarily lower the arm in a smooth and continuous fashion, and is highly suggestive of a complete rotator cuff tear.[23,24]

Multiple regional tests exist to determine the tissue injured and the level of apprehension or instability. Some of the most commonly used tests in the clinical setting are listed in **Table 2** .[23–25]

OUTCOME MEASURES

Clinicians are encouraged to consider the use of clinical outcome measures to establish objective data in each patient and to subsequently use that data to monitor treatment response.

For example, the Disabilities of the Arm, Shoulder, and Hand (DASH) questionnaire, is a 30-item questionnaire that assesses the ability of a patient to perform certain upper extremity activities.[29] It is a self-report questionnaire with which patients can rate difficulty and interference with daily life, and self-care skills.

In addition to the DASH questionnaire, there are multiple practical, well-validated, and easy-to-administer outcome measures, such as the Functional Reach Test, the 6-Minute Walk Test, and the Timed Up-and-Go Test.

All these tests can be performed fairly quickly in the clinical setting. They may provide invaluable information in monitoring treatment response and identifying needed rehabilitation and supporting resources for older adults.

Once a diagnosis is reached and a standard medical treatment plan has been delineated, the rehabilitation process can begin.

ADDRESSING AND DOCUMENTING THE NEED FOR PHYSICAL REHABILITATION

It is important to remember that older adults with regional rheumatic disorders may need additional care, beyond standard medical treatment, to achieve and maintain an optimal level of functioning. Many older adults have multiple comorbidities and may be affected by polypharmacy. Therefore, awareness and the use of nonpharmacologic therapies are crucial. Physical rehabilitation is an important adjunct to pharmacologic treatment in many patients.[17]

Table 2
Common special tests for regional rheumatic disorders

Body Region	Special Tests
Shoulder	• Speed test for biceps tendinitis • Yergason test for bicipital tendon instability • Neer-Walsh impingement test for rotator cuff tendinitis
Elbow	• Cozen test for lateral epicondylitis
Wrist and hand	• Finkelstein test for de Quervain tenosynovitis
Hip	• Thomas test • Ober test • Patrick test
Knees	• Lachman test • McMurray test • Valgus and varus stress test
Ankles	• Anterior drawer test • Thompson test

Data from O'Sullivan SB, Schmitz TJ, Fulk GD. Physical rehabilitation. Philadelphia: F.A. Davis Co.; 2014; and Richards S, Cristian A. The role of the physical therapist in the care of the older adult. Clin Geriatr Med 2006;22(2):269–79.

THE PHILOSOPHY OF PHYSICAL REHABILITATION

Maintaining functional independence is a key indicator of life satisfaction in older adults.[16] In physical rehabilitation, functioning represents both the starting point and the outcome of patient/client management. Traditional biomedical models of health care often focus solely on the diagnosis and treatment of underlying disease. In contrast, physical rehabilitation philosophy considers the biopsychosocial model of health care. The broad goal is to treat the whole person, rather than focus on a singular medical problem. Biological, psychological, and social factors all play important roles in human functioning. These factors account for the day-to-day variation in function of individuals as well as functional differences between individuals with similar disease severity.[30]

The World Health Organization's International Classification of Function (ICF; **Fig. 4**) is based on the biopsychosocial model and provides clinicians with a unified, standard language and framework for capturing how people with health conditions function in their daily lives. Using the ICF's terminology, health conditions cause impairments in body structure and function; these impairments affect activity and ultimately inhibit societal participation.[31] Rehabilitation professionals are challenged to think holistically about patient care needs, including systematically identifying specific impairments, activity limitations, and participation restrictions, in conjunction with personal and environmental contextual factors.

GENERAL CONSIDERATIONS IN GERIATRIC REHABILITATION

Although the fundamental principles of physical rehabilitation are similar regardless of the patient's age, there are unique features and considerations in the management of older adults that can greatly improve outcomes.[32]

Aging is a heterogeneous process

With increasing age, older adults become increasingly dissimilar, and these dissimilarities cannot be attributed to age alone.[32] Understanding the heterogeneous nature of

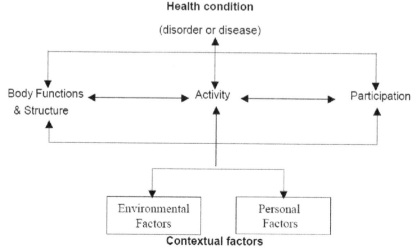

Fig. 4. ICF. (*From* WHO. Towards a common language for functioning, disability and health: ICF.Geneva: World Health Organization; 2002. p. 9, with permission.)

the older population is crucial to the success of any rehabilitation plan of care. Clinicians must keep in mind that stereotypical information, although helpful in understanding older people as a global population, may not fit any individual situation.[33,34]

Older Adults Commonly Have Multiple Chronic Conditions

More than two-thirds of older Americans have 2 or more chronic conditions and 14% have 6 or more.[30] Furthermore, acute illnesses can be superimposed on these chronic conditions, which makes rehabilitation management complex and challenging. Therefore, a multidisciplinary approach is important in the delivery of geriatric rehabilitative services. Multidisciplinary team management assists in ensuring that patients receive comprehensive evaluations and care for the primary health condition and all associated comorbidities.[31]

Older Adults Have Unique Psychosocial Needs

Adults face many different transitions throughout life. In the case of older adults, many of these transitions are characterized by physical, psychological, social, and economic loss. To provide successful rehabilitative services, clinicians must comprehensively consider the psychosocial factors that may influence (both positively and negatively) the client's participation in rehabilitation, and then place the physical findings in the context of the older adult's psychosocial environment.

Physical Rehabilitation Efforts Should Focus On Function

Because maintaining functional independence is a key indicator of life satisfaction in older adults,[16] the goal of physical rehabilitation should be to restore and maintain each individual's highest level of desired function and independence within that individual's environment. Rehabilitation professionals should be able to, without bias, creatively address the client's functional goals while incorporating clinical evidence and expertise.[32]

THE PLAN OF CARE

Once the older adult's impairments and functional limitations have been identified, a rehabilitation plan of care is designed by the clinician. The plan of care delineates specific goals and expected outcomes, specific interventions, intervention frequency, and the estimated duration of care. The plan of care is not static. Instead, it is an iterative process that evolves over the course of care.[12] It is important to reiterate that older adults frequently have multiple chronic diseases that affect multiple body systems, including the cardiovascular, pulmonary, neuromuscular, integumentary, renal, and gastrointestinal systems.[13] Reevaluation of the individual's current health status and how it affects the patient's physical functioning and ability to participate in rehabilitation is a vital recursive process. Clinicians also use this information to identify specific precautions that need to be followed during treatment[14] and to determine whether referral to another provider is indicated.[12]

Goal Setting

The development of specific goals for older adults with regional rheumatic disorders is based on the general goals presented in **Table 3** . The specific goals identified for each patient depend on the specific disorder, the severity of the disorder, the overall clinical presentation, and the patient's preferences.[13] Clinicians must remember that rehabilitation is active work done by the patient, and not to the patient. Therefore, older adults' choices, desires, preferences, and expectations must be placed at

Table 3	
General goals and outcomes for individuals with regional rheumatic disorders	
Impact of impairments in body structures/ functions is reduced	• Pain is decreased • ROM of all joints is maximized and sufficient for functional activities • Muscle activation and strength are maximized and sufficient for functional activities • Joint stability is maximized and biomechanical stresses on all affected joints are decreased; deformity prevented • Endurance is increased for all functional activities and desired recreational activities
Ability to perform activities is improved	• Independence in ADL is promoted, including dressing, transfers, and self-care • Efficiency and safety of gait pattern and balance are improved • Patterns of adequate physical activity or exercise to maintain or improve MSK and cardiovascular fitness and general health are established
Health status and quality of life are improved	Patient, family, and caregivers are educated to promote the individual's capacity for self-management

Abbreviation: ADL, activities of daily living.

Data from World Health Organization. Towards a common language for functioning, disability and health: ICF. Geneva: World Health Organization; 2002.

the center of the process, and it is clear that the patient must be part of the goal-setting process. The presence of psychological disorders and/or cognitive dysfunction may limit the collaborative process. However, having the opportunity to provide input on even the smallest aspects of the plan of care can provide motivation for older adults.[35] It is the clinician's responsibility to ensure that the goals are realistic, objective, measurable, and time limited. In addition, goals and expected outcomes should be reviewed with the patient at regular intervals and modified as necessary.[12]

NONINVASIVE PROCEDURAL INTERVENTIONS

Rehabilitation professionals use information gathered through the examination to select interventions best suited to meet the individual's needs.[12] The selection of interventions may be affected by psychosocial factors such as financial resources, social support, living environment, and the older adult's interests. To optimize this process, the intervention plan should be established and managed in collaboration with the older adult whenever possible. This collaboration is an important step toward empowering older adults to take responsibility for their own recovery.[35]

Noninvasive procedural interventions for older adults with regional rheumatic disorders focus on the following areas (**Table 4**):

- Pain relief (thermal agents, electrotherapy, protective and supportive devices)
- Joint range of motion/flexibility
- Strengthening exercises
- Aerobic conditioning
- Functional training
- Aquatic exercise

Table 4
Procedural interventions for older adults with regional rheumatic disorders

Pain Relief[a]	*Thermal Agents* • Includes superficial heating modalities (eg, moist hot packs, paraffin wax, Fluidotherapy), deep heating modalities (eg, ultrasonography, diathermy), and cryotherapy (eg, cold packs, ice massage, cold therapy machines) • Literature on the efficacy of thermal agents on pain in older adults is limited; however, they are frequently used clinically and in self-management of chronic pain among older adults[17,35] • Note contraindication/precautions for use • Patient education on appropriate home use is essential because these modalities carry a risk of injury[17] *TENS* • Literature on the efficacy of TENS is inconclusive, particularly for chronic pain.[17,35,36] However, patients using TENS have reported distraction from pain resulting in positive benefits such as medication reduction, better function, psychological benefits, and better rest[37] • There is evidence that both conventional (high-frequency) and burst-mode TENS result in short-term pain relief in older adults with chronic pain. However, patients reported conventional TENS as more comfortable[38] • Note contraindication/precautions for use • Determining treatment parameters and educating patients/caregivers on appropriate use is essential, because this may influence effectiveness[39] *Protective/Supportive Devices* • These devices may assist in decreasing pain and increasing function by supporting and protecting weak, fragile, or unbalanced muscles and joints[35] • Splinting may help preserve function by holding joints in a proper position and preventing tissue shortening or contracture[40] • Gait aids can assist with load transfer across joints[17] • Appropriate footwear and shoe orthotics may decrease loads across lower extremity joints and improve lower extremity alignment[17] • Decisions regarding use should be individualized based on information gained in the examination. Appropriate device selection and measurements are important in order to improve efficiency.[35] Cognition and coordination also influence the selection process[33]
ROM/Flexibility	• Static stretching is preferred to dynamic stretching for lengthening muscle and collagen tissue[17] • Because of tissue extensibility changes in older adults, a 60-s hold is preferred to achieve long-term effects[41] • Stretching exercises performed regularly, 5–7 d/wk, seem to be most effective[41] • Stretching programs should be individualized based on the specific disorder and the patient's feedback regarding pain • Stretching exercises in the presence of joint instability are contraindicated[17]
Strengthening	• Well-designed strengthening programs improve function; decrease impact of chronic disease; and improve balance, coordination, speed of movement, and overall mobility. However, strength training is often underused and undermanaged for older adults[17] • Strengthening programs should be progressive and individualized based on the specific disorder and the patient's feedback regarding pain

(continued on next page)

Table 4 (continued)	
	• High-intensity resistance training (80% of 1-repetition max) improves strength and function greater than low-intensity training and is safe when done properly[42] • Eccentric training increases strength and function with less cardiovascular stress, especially in those who are deconditioned[42] • Power training (plyometrics) can complement traditional training to improve speed and the ability to perform ADLs[42,43] • Caution should be taken to ensure that older adults maintain proper form and avoid breath holding. It is recommended that high-intensity resistance training be done under the direct supervision of a physical therapist[17]
Aerobic Conditioning	• Involves continuous, rhythmic movement using large muscle groups • Increases the body's capacity to absorb, deliver, and use oxygen, thus improving the older adult's ability to complete desired activities without becoming fatigued[17] • Older adults' physical impairments, functional deficits, and personal goals need to be considered when selecting the mode of exercise. The mode should require little skill or extra equipment • Be aware of any contraindication/precautions for aerobic exercise. Patients with undiagnosed or poorly managed cardiovascular symptoms should be referred for a medical evaluation before commencing aerobic conditioning *Aquatic Exercise* • A safe and beneficial alternative for older adults who cannot tolerate the stresses of land-based exercises because of pain or instability.[17,42,44] • Should be used in conjunction with land-based therapy for functional carryover[17,42,44] • Individuals need to be able to move safely into and out of the pool and maneuver around the pool area[17] • May have an additional benefit of social support through group classes[42] • Contraindicated for individuals with incontinence, open wounds, or allergies to the chemicals in pool water. Other precautions/contraindications are the same as with any form of aerobic activity[17]
Functional Training	• Includes training in basic ADL (eg, feeding, dressing, self-care), functional mobility tasks (eg, bed mobility, transferring, gait), and instrumental ADL (eg, house chores, grocery shopping). Tasks targeted depend on the older adult's level of function • Challenges individuals to use multiple joints through multiple axes of motion while incorporating body weight and balance • Has been shown to be more effective at improving functional task performance than resistance exercises alone[45] and flexibility exercises alone[46] • Should be performed in environments that are similar to those regularly encountered by the client[47,48] • Rehabilitation professionals may choose to use assistive devices/adaptive equipment to promote safety and maximize independence

Abbreviation: TENS, transcutaneous electrical nerve stimulation.

[a] These passive interventions should be used sparingly in conjunction with more active, functional interventions.[35]

Data from Refs.[17,33,35–37,39–47]

PATIENT EDUCATION

Patient education is an essential component of health care. The patient (and/or care-giver) needs to take personal control over the prevention and management of the condition. However, myths concerning learning in the later years often negatively influence the perception of older adult's ability to learn new material. There is evidence of age-related declines in attentiveness, concentration, performance, short-term memory, and speed of learning. However, older adults, barring certain diseases, retain the ability to learn and understand well into late life. To compensate for age-related changes, a well-planned approach to instruction is necessary.[33] Rehabilitation professionals gain information about the older individual's learning style and learning capabilities, and then adapt instructional sessions to enhance the learning process.

For older adults with regional rheumatic disorders, education on joint protection, energy conservation, and environmental adaptations is essential, because these are key components of self-management.

Joint Protection

Regional rheumatic disorders may render the involved joint weak and unstable; therefore, education on how to protect the joints is necessary. General joint protection principles include[13]:

- Respect pain
- Balance rest with activity
- Exercise in a pain-free range
- Avoid maintaining the joint in flexion for a prolonged period of time
- Use large, strong joints
- Use adaptive equipment/assistive devices as needed

Energy Conservation

Energy conservation techniques are particularly useful for older adults who may have comorbidities resulting in impaired aerobic capacity. By conserving energy, older adults may be able to do more of the activities they enjoy with less pain and fatigue, in addition to completing their activities of daily living. These strategies include[32]:

- Modifying activities (eg, sitting vs standing)
- Organizing activities to reduce redundancy of movement (eg, organizing household chores to reduce the number of times the stairs must be negotiated)
- Prioritizing tasks according to importance
- Delegating tasks to other individuals as appropriate

Environmental Adaptations

Normal age-related changes can affect older adults' ability to function safely in their home environments. The addition of a regional rheumatic disorder further complicates the situation. Adjustments to the older adult's existing environment can reduce the risk of falling,[49] enhance independence, and improve quality of life. Most environmental adaptations can be divided into 3 categories:

1. Removing hazards (eg, removing clutter, cords, throw rugs; placing frequently used items within reach)
2. Providing appropriate lighting (eg, using night lights, preventing excessive glare)
3. Installing adaptive equipment (eg, handrails on both sides of a staircase, grab bars in the bathroom, tub bench/elevated toilet seat in the bathroom)

Rehabilitation professionals can provide guidance on which adaptations are needed and assist older adults (or caregivers) in prioritizing the needed changes.

INVASIVE PHYSIATRIC INTERVENTIONS

If patients fail to improve with the noninvasive therapies described earlier, enteral or topical medications and/or invasive interventions may be recommended.

Acupuncture/Dry Needling

Acupuncture and/or dry needling (ADN) are therapies that are commonly performed by physiatrists, physical therapists, and other practitioners. Pain is the most common diagnosis for which acupuncture is prescribed in a physiatric practice.[50] Reported benefits of ADN include analgesia, decreased swelling/edema, improved range of motion, and improved mood/affect. There is minimal risk with ADN and few contraindications other than infection at the site of pin insertion.[51]

Intra-articular Injections

Joint injections are performed either by palpation (using anatomic landmarks), with fluoroscopy, or increasingly with US guidance. Joint aspiration confirms intra-articular placement of the needle. Localization of some joints can be challenging and many physicians prefer image-based guidance for these procedures[52] (**Fig. 5**).

Intra-articular injections (IAI) are commonly recommended for symptomatic relief. The most commonly recommended agents for IAI are corticosteroids or viscoagents (hyaluronic acid [HA]) but increasingly IAI of so-called regenerative agents, including blood-derived products (platelet-rich plasma [PRP]) or prolotherapy, are offered to patients.[53]

Viscohyaluronic Acid

Several HA products are US Food and Drug Administration approved in the United States, and all are produced from in-vitro bacterial fermentation or from harvested combs of roosters. HA injection reportedly restores the viscoelastic properties of dysfunctional synovial fluids, and may have a protective effect on hyaline cartilage and a disease-modifying effect for rheumatoid arthritis.[54] Given the heterogeneity of

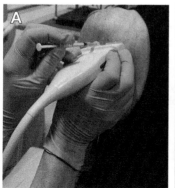
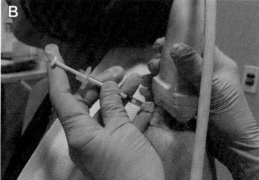

Fig. 5. (A) US-guided glenohumeral joint injection. (B) US-guided acromioclavicular joint injection.

products, trial design, and patients, it is not surprising that studies report a range of benefits from HA injections.[55]

Regenerative Injections

Regenerative joint injections with PRP or prolotherapy are gaining acceptance by clinicians and patients and are an effective alternative to traditional agents. Although an increasing body of literature supports the efficacy of these agents, they are generally considered complementary or alternative therapies and are therefore not covered by third-party payers.

Prolotherapy

Prolotherapy refers to the injection of hypertonic dextrose solutions or, less commonly, morrhuate sodium into joints; other MSK structures, such as tendons; and/or for other pain conditions.[51,56] The reported mechanism of action of prolotherapy is promotion of enhanced healing and tissue repair in a wide variety of MSK tissues, including tendons, muscle, ligaments, and joint cartilage with the formation of new collagen fibers.[57]

Platelet-rich Plasma

PRP injections are reported to benefit patients with osteoarthritis, cartilage damage, epicondylosis, tendinosis, and other MSK conditions. PRP is an injectate derived from the platelet layer of autologous blood. Although there is a growing body of evidence that supports the safety and efficacy of PRP for the treatment of a wide variety of MSK conditions, additional high-quality placebo-controlled trials are needed.[58-60]

Soft Tissue Injections

Injection therapy is recommended for a wide variety of MSK soft tissue conditions, including myofascial pain conditions, trigger points, tendinopathies, epicondylosis, and muscle or ligament injuries. Injectate options include a wide variety of drugs/ agents, including local anesthetics, corticosteroids, prolotherapy, PRP, botulinum toxins, and phenol thers.[51,61] To select the most appropriate agent for each patients, clinicians must be familiar with the potential benefits and risks of each product. A full review of the other agents is beyond the scope of this article and readers are referred to reviews on this topic.[51,56,61]

Ultrasonography-guided Needle Fenestration/Tenotomy

US-guided percutaneous needle fenestration or tenotomy is recommended as an alternative to surgery for refractory chronic tendinopathies.[62,63] The procedure involves repeatedly passing the needle through the area of degeneration, leading to local inflammation, bleeding, inflammation, and the release of growth factors. Commonly treated areas include the elbow, patella, Achilles, and less commonly the hip or pubic symphysis. US-guided tenotomy combined with PRP injections have also been reported.[64] Studies show few complications and promising results.[63]

FUTURE RESEARCH CONSIDERATIONS

The number of older adults with and without regional rheumatic disorders will continue to grow over the next few decades. In order to optimize patients' functional independence for as long as feasible, it is important to gain an understanding of the disease process and its effects superimposed on the normal aging processes. Research topics to consider are listed in **Box 4**.

Box 4
Future research topics to consider

- Optimizing the classification, nomenclature, and taxonomy of regional rheumatic disorders in older adults.
- Completing a comprehensive epidemiologic study of regional rheumatic disorders in older adults.
- Pursuing basic science research on soft tissues wear and tear.
- Identifying clinical and diagnostic biomarkers for regional rheumatic disorders in older adults.
- Studying the impact of comprehensive rehabilitation interventions in this population in relation to cost and function.
- Systematic investigation of regenerative procedures and injections.
- Studying the safety and efficacy of image-guided versus blind injection procedures.

REFERENCES

1. Picavet HSJ, Hazes JMW. Prevalence of self reported musculoskeletal diseases is high. Ann Rheum Dis 2003;62:644–50.
2. Van Lankveld W, Goossens J, Franssen M. The gerontorheumatology outpatient service: toward the international classification of function-based health care provision for the elderly with musculoskeletal conditions: geriatric rheumatology: a comprehensive approach. Springer Science + Business Media; 2011. p. 85–91.
3. Herr KA, Garand L. Assessment and measurement of pain in older adults. Pain Med 2007;8(7):585–601.
4. Borsheski R, Johnson QL. Pain management in the geriatric population. Mo Med 2014;111(6):508–11.
5. Auret K, Schug SA. Underutilisation of opioids in elderly patients with chronic pain. Drugs Aging 2005;22(8):641–54.
6. Ahmed MS, Matsumura B, Cristian A. Age-related changes in muscles and joints. Aging with a disability. Phys Med Rehabil Clin N Am 2005;16(1):16–39.
7. Tummala MK, Taubb DD, Ershler WB. Clinical immunology: immune senescence and the acquired immune deficiency of aging. In: Fillit HM, Rockwood K, Woodhouse K, editors. Brocklehurst's textbook of geriatric medicine and gerontology. 7th Edition. Philadelphia: Saunders- Elsevier; 2010. p. 83–6.
8. de Lateur BJ. Rehabilitative strategies. Gonzalez-Fernandez M, Friedman JD, editors. Physical medicine and rehabilitation pocket companion. New York: Demos Medical; p. 1–3.
9. Lipsky P, Cush J. Approach to articular and musculoskeletal disorders. In: Fauci AS, editor. Harrison's rheumatology. McGraw-Hill; 2006. p. 227–39.
10. Speed C. Classification of soft tissue disorders: soft tissue rheumatology. Oxford University Press; 2004. p. 141–5.
11. Biundo J Jr. Musculoskeletal signs and symptoms D. Regional rheumatic pain syndromes. In: Klippel JH, et al, editors. Primer on the rheumatic diseases. 13th edition. Springer; 2008. p. 68–86.
12. Guide to physical therapist practice 3.0. Alexandria (VA): American Physical Therapy Association; 2014. Available at: http://guidetoptpractice.apta.org. Accessed February 8, 2016.

13. O'Sullivan SB, Schmitz TJ, Fulk GD. Physical rehabilitation. Philadelphia: FA Davis; 2014.
14. Richards S, Cristian A. The role of the physical therapist in the care of the older adult. Clin Geriatr Med 2006;22(2):269–79.
15. Bloch RM. Geriatric rehabilitation. In: Braddom RL, et al, editors. Physical medicine and rehabilitation. 4th Edition. Elsevier; 2007. p. 1419–37.
16. Federal Interagency Forum on Aging-Related Statistics. Older Americans 2012: key indicators of well-being. Washington, DC: US Government Printing Office; 2012.
17. Vlieland TPV. Multidisciplinary team care and outcomes in rheumatoid arthritis. Curr Opin Rheumatol 2004;16(2):153–6.
18. Adler RS, Finzel KC. The complementary roles of MR imaging and ultrasound of tendons. Radiol Clin North Am 2005;43:771–807, ix.
19. Grassi W, Lamanna G, Farina A, et al. Sonographic imaging of normal and osteoarthritic cartilage. Semin Arthritis Rheum 1999;28:398–403.
20. Mathew AJ, Danda D, Conaghan PG. MRI and ultrasound in rheumatoid arthritis. Curr Opin Rheumatol 2016;28(3):323–9.
21. Smith J, Finnoff JT. Diagnostic and interventional musculoskeletal ultrasound: part 1. Fundamentals. PM R 2009;1(1):64–75.
22. Smith J, Finnoff JT. Diagnostic and interventional musculoskeletal ultrasound: part 2. Clinical applications. PM R 2009;1(2):162–77.
23. Finnoff JT. Musculoskeletal disorders of the upper limb. In: Braddon RL, et al, editors. Physical medicine and rehabilitation. 4th edition. Elsevier; 2007. p. 817–42.
24. Finnoff JT. Musculoskeletal disorders of the upper limb. In: Hazzard WR, Halter JB, editors. Hazzard's geriatric medicine and gerontology. New York: McGraw-Hill Medical; 2009.
25. Hansen PA, Willick SE. Musculoskeletal disorders of the lower limb. In: Braddon RL, et al, editors. Physical medicine and rehabilitation. 4th edition. Elsevier; 2007. p. 843–70.
26. Frontera, WR., Silver, JK., Rizzo Jr, TD. Essentials of physical medicine and rehabilitation, musculoskeletal disorders, pain and rehabilitation. 2nd Edition. Saunders.
27. Griffin LY. Essentials of musculoskeletal care. 3rd Edition. AAOS; 2005.
28. Gilliland BC. Periarticular disorders of the extremities. Fauci AS. Harrison's rheumatology. 2006. p. 299–302.
29. Beaton DE, Katz JN, Fossel AH, et al. Measuring the whole or the parts? Validity, reliability, and responsiveness of the Disabilities of the Arm, Shoulder and Hand outcome measure in different regions of the upper extremity. J Hand Ther 2001;14(2):128–46.
30. Wade D. Rehabilitation - a new approach. Part two: the underlying theories. Clin Rehabil 2015;29(12):1145–54.
31. Stott D, Quinn T. Principles of rehabilitation of older people. Medicine 2013;41(1):1–4.
32. Guccione A, Wong R, Avers D. Geriatric physical therapy. 3rd Edition. St Louis (MO): Mosby; 2012.
33. Saxon SV, Etten MJ, Perkins EA. Physical change and aging: a guide for the helping professions. 6th edition. New York: Springer Publishing Company; 2014.
34. Centers for Medicare and Medicaid Services. Chronic conditions among Medicare beneficiaries, chartbook, 2012 Edition. Baltimore (MD): Centers for Medicare and Medicaid Services; 2012.
35. Drench ME, Noonan A, Sharby N, et al. Psychosocial aspects of health care. 3rd edition. Upper Saddle River (NJ): Pearson Education; 2012.

36. Edeer AO, Tuna H. Management of chronic musculoskeletal pain in the elderly: dilemmas and remedies. INTECH Open Access Publisher; 2012.
37. Abdulla A, Adams N, Bone M, et al. Guidance on the management of pain in older people. Age Ageing 2013;42(Suppl 1):i1–57.
38. Gladwell PW, Badlan K, Cramp F, et al. Direct and indirect benefits reported by users of transcutaneous electrical nerve stimulation for chronic musculoskeletal pain: qualitative exploration using patient interviews. Phys Ther 2015;95(11): 1518–28.
39. Barr J, Weissenbuehler S, Cleary C. Effectiveness and comfort of transcutaneous electrical nerve stimulation for older persons with chronic pain. J Geriatr Phys Ther 2004;27:93–9.
40. Bennett MI, Hughes N, Johnson MI. Methodological quality in randomised controlled trials of transcutaneous electric nerve stimulation for pain: low fidelity may explain negative findings. Pain 2011;152:1226–32.
41. Radomski MV, Trombly CA. Occupational therapy for physical dysfunction. Philadelphia: Wolters Kluwer Health; 2014.
42. Feland JB, Myrer JW, Schulthies SS, et al. The effect of duration of stretching of the hamstring muscle group for increasing range of motion in people aged 65 years and older. Phys Ther 2001;81:1110–7.
43. Kemmis K. The aging musculoskeletal system. Focus: physical therapist practice in geriatrics. Academy of Geriatric Physical Therapy 2011;1:1–31.
44. Cuoco A, Callahan DM, Sayers S, et al. Impact of muscle power and force on gait speed in disabled older men and women. J Gerontol A Biol Sci Med Sci 2004; 59(11):1200–6.
45. Takeshima N, Rogers ME, Watanabe E, et al. Water-based exercise improves health-related aspects of fitness in older women. Med Sci Sports Exerc 2002; 33:544–51.
46. de Vreede PL, Samson MM, van Meeteren NL, et al. Functional-task exercise versus resistance strength exercise to improve daily function in older women: a randomized, controlled trial. J Am Geriatr Soc 2005;53:2–10.
47. Alexander N, Galecki AT, Grenier ML, et al. Task-specific resistance training to improve the ability of activities of daily living-impaired older adults to rise from a bed and from a chair. J Am Geriatr Soc 2001;49(11):1418–27.
48. Jones CJ, Rose D. Physical activity instruction of older adults. Champaign (IL): Human Kinetics; 2005.
49. Gillespie LD, Robertson MC, Gillespie WJ, et al. Interventions for preventing falls in older people living in the community. Cochrane Database Syst Rev 2012;(9):CD007146.
50. Tough EA, White AR, Cummings TM, et al. Acupuncture and dry needling in the management of myofascial trigger point pain: a systematic review and meta-analysis of randomized controlled trials. Eur J Pain 2009;13:3–10.
51. Singh V, Trescot A, Nishio I. Injections for chronic pain. Phys Med Rehabil Clin N Am 2015;26(2):249–61.
52. Davisdon J, Jayaraman S. Guided interventions in musculoskeletal ultrasound: what's the evidence? Clin Radiol 2011;66(2):140–52.
53. Rabago D, Zgierska A, Fortney L, et al. Hypertonic dextrose injections (prolotherapy) for knee osteoarthritis: results of a single-arm uncontrolled study with 1-year follow-up. J Altern Complement Med 2012;18(4):408–14.
54. Ayhan E, Kesmezacar H, Akgun S. Intraarticular injections (corticosteroid, hyaluronic acid, platelet rich plasma) for the knee osteoarthritis. World J Orthop 2014;5(3):351–61.

55. Bannuru RR, Natov NS, Dasi UR, et al. Therapeutic trajectory following intra-articular hyaluronic acid injection in knee osteoarthritis–meta-analysis. Osteoarthritis Cartilage 2011;19:611–9.

56. Fullerton BD, Reeves KD. Ultrasonography in regenerative injection (prolotherapy) using dextrose, platelet-rich plasma, and other injectants. Phys Med Rehabil Clin N Am 2010;21(3):585–605.

57. Park J, Song I, Lee J, et al. Ultrasonographic findings of healing of torn tendon in the patients with lateral epicondylitis after prolotherapy. J Korean Soc Med Ultrasonography 2003;22(3):177–83.

58. Palacio EP, Schiavetti RR, Kanematsu M, et al. Effects of platelet-rich plasma on lateral epicondylitis of the elbow: prospective randomized controlled trial. Rev Bras Ortop 2016;51(1):90–5.

59. Vannini F, Di Matteo B, Filardo G. Platelet-rich plasma to treat ankle cartilage pathology - from translational potential to clinical evidence: a systematic review. J Exp Orthop 2015;2(1):2.

60. Lai PL, Stitik TP, Foye PM, et al. Use of platelet-rich plasma in intra-articular knee injections for osteoarthritis: a systematic review. PM R 2015;7(6):637–48.

61. Alter K, Wilson N. Botulinum toxin therapy for musculoskeletal conditions. In: Botulinum toxin injection manual. New York: Demos Medical Publishing; 2014. p. 260–84.

62. Jacobson JA, Rubin J, Yablon CM, et al. Ultrasound-guided fenestration of tendons about the hip and pelvis: clinical outcomes. J Ultrasound Med 2015; 34(11):2029–35.

63. Housner JA, Jacobson JA, Misko R. Sonographically guided percutaneous needle tenotomy for the treatment of chronic tendinosis. J Ultrasound Med 2009; 28(9):1187–92.

64. Finnoff JT, Fowler SP, Lai JK, et al. Treatment of chronic tendinopathy with ultrasound-guided needle tenotomy and platelet-rich plasma injection. PM R 2011;3(10):900–11.

Rheumatologic Manifestations of Malignancy

Mandana Hashefi, MD

KEYWORDS

- Musculoskeletal • Malignancy • Mimics • Paraneoplastic • Lymphoma
- Pitting edema • Fasciitis • Autoimmune

KEY POINTS

- Autoimmune conditions and their treatments may be associated with an increased risk of certain malignancies.
- The lack of response to conventional treatment of a rheumatic syndrome (such as polymyalgia rheumatica or inflammatory polyarthritis) should raise the suspicion for a paraneoplastic etiology.
- Conditions such as palmar fasciitis with polyarthritis, hypertrophic osteoarthropathy, multicentric reticulohistiocytosis, and dermatomyositis have well-documented evidence for association with underlying malignancy.
- A higher incidence of non-Hodgkin's lymphoma and other hematologic and lymphoproliferative diseases is seen in patients with primary Sjögren's syndrome, systemic sclerosis, rheumatoid arthritis, and lupus, among others.

INTRODUCTION

Kankeleit[1] noted one of the earliest associations between cancer and polymyositis in 1916. Since then, a variety of clinical and epidemiologic associations between musculoskeletal symptoms and underlying malignancies have been described. However, determining causality between these conditions and malignancy remains challenging.

Certain malignancies occur with higher incidence in patients with autoimmune disorders. Mechanistically, this may relate to malignant transformation that can occur as a result of immune dysregulation in the later phase of certain autoimmune conditions. For example, non-Hodgkin's lymphomas (NHLs) are reported with higher frequency in patients with primary Sjögren's syndrome, rheumatoid arthritis (RA), and possibly in systemic lupus erythematosus (SLE).[2]

Disclosure Statement: The author has nothing to disclose.
Division of Rheumatology, George Washington University, 2300, M Street, Northwest, Suite: 3-307, Washington, DC 20037, USA
E-mail address: mhashefi@mfa.gwu.edu

Many clinical presentations mimic rheumatologic conditions, which, in reality, are direct signs of the musculoskeletal spread of the underlying cancer or a paraneoplastic syndrome associated with it. These paraneoplastic rheumatic syndromes are not directly caused by local or distant spread of the tumor but are actually induced through a complex interaction of humoral and cytotoxic immune mechanisms, autocrine and paracrine mediators, and signaling pathways.

Certain conditions, such as hypertrophic osteoarthropathy (HOA), dermatomyositis, and palmar fasciitis with polyarthritis have well-documented associations with cancer. However, a growing body of literature describes other conditions, including but not limited to, remitting seronegative symmetric synovitis with pitting edema (RS3PE), carcinogenic polyarthritis, multicentric reticulohistiocytosis (MRH), leukocytoclastic vasculitis (LCV), scleroderma and the scleroderma mimics, eosinophilic fasciitis, and erythromelalgia, which will be further discussed below.

It is difficult at times to discern association from coincidence, as some of these associations are merely based on case reports or small series. Another limitation is that some reports are subject to a "Berkson's bias," which occurs when patients, but not controls, are drawn from a hospital referral population. In this situation, the possibility of recognition of a hospitalized patient with both a primary rheumatic disorder and malignancy is much higher than for a patient with a rheumatic disorder alone. Finally, some reported associations are based on standardized incidence ratios (SIRs) and odds ratios, which reflect correlation between 2 disorders and not necessarily causality.[3]

In 1965, Sir Austin Bradford Hill proposed criteria to guide establishing an argument for causation.[4] These criteria may be used to determine if a given rheumatic condition can be attributed to the presence of an underlying malignancy. The summary of Bradford Hill's criteria are as follows: strength of association between the causative agent and the outcome, temporal sequence of the 2 conditions, consistency of results even when different methodology is used, theoretic plausibility, coherence (which means if the association makes theoretic sense), specificity in the causes, dose-response relationship, experimental evidence, and similar evidence from analogous conditions.[5]

The emphasis of this article is to raise awareness of those musculoskeletal conditions that should alert the clinician to a search for an occult malignancy. However, a comprehensive review of the primary and metastatic tumors of the musculoskeletal system is beyond the scope of this report.

CLINICAL CLUES FOR PRESENCE OF AN OCCULT MALIGNANCY

Several features can raise suspicion for the presence of an occult malignancy in an older patient with musculoskeletal complaints. Some of these include personal or family history of malignancy, prior exposure to carcinogenic medications or environmental pollutants, constitutional symptoms, unusual clinical picture for the rheumatic syndrome, and atypical or no response to conventional therapy.

There are other alarming presentations that may also trigger more intense search for occult malignancy, such as sudden-onset asymmetric polyarthritis presenting in the elderly, rheumatoid arthritis with monoclonal gammopathy, Sjögren's syndrome with increasing globulin-albumin gap, hypertrophic osteoarthropathy, dermatomyositis, polymyalgia rheumatica unresponsive to prednisone therapy, eosinophilic fasciitis poorly responsive to corticosteroid therapy, erythema nodosum lasting more than 6 months, and the new onset of Raynaud's phenomenon or cutaneous leukocytoclastic vasculitis after age 50 years.[6]

SPECTRUM OF RHEUMATOLOGIC MANIFESTATIONS OF MALIGNANCIES

The musculoskeletal manifestations of malignancy can be caused by several underlying conditions. Symptoms may result from involvement of the bone, joint, muscles, or associated structures by the primary or metastatic tumors. Also some specific autoimmune rheumatologic conditions are inherently associated with increased risk of malignancies. In addition, a variety of other factors, such as altered immune responses from treatment with immunosuppressive and antineoplastic medications, can contribute to development of rheumatologic manifestations in cancer patients.

Primary or Metastatic Tumors Involving the Bone, Joint, Muscles, or Associated Structures

Musculoskeletal structure including bones, articular cartilage, and synovium as well as muscles and other periarticular structures can become directly involved by a variety of benign or malignant neoplastic conditions. Primary malignant bone tumors, although uncommon, can cause significant cancer-related morbidity and mortality, particularly among younger people. Approximately 3300 primary malignant bone tumors are diagnosed annually in the United States, resulting in 1490 deaths each year. This does not include the extensive bone involvement that can be seen with hematologic malignancies such as multiple myeloma, leukemia, and lymphomas. The cumulative annual incidence for these latter neoplasms is approximately 172,000 cases in the United States alone.[7]

The World Health Organization Classification of Tumors of Soft Tissue and Bone, published in 2013, categorizes these tumors based on the tissue of origin, regardless of the malignant or benign nature of the tumor. The categories described in this classification include chondrogenic, osteogenic, fibrogenic, and fibrohistiocytic tumors as well as Ewing sarcoma; hematopoietic neoplasms; osteoclastic giant cell–rich tumors; notochondral, vascular, myogenic, lipogenic, and epithelial tumors; tumors of undefined neoplastic nature; and undifferentiated high-grade pleomorphic sarcomas.[8] Some tumors have a predilection for certain joints. As an example, pigmented villonodular synovitis, synovial hemangioma, synovial osteochondromatosis, and lipomatosis arborescens are a few of the benign tumors occurring in larger joints such as the knees. The primary malignant intra-articular knee lesions also include synovial sarcoma and synovial chondrosarcoma.

Certain cancers such as lung, breast, and prostate have a tendency to metastasize to bone. Breast cancer metastases are usually osteolytic with some reactive osteoblastic activity, whereas prostate cancer metastatic lesions are usually osteoblastic presenting with elevated alkaline phosphatase and osteocalcin bone turnover markers.[9] Several other malignancies can spread to the bone. These metastatic lesions may be categorized as primarily osteolytic (eg, renal cell carcinoma, multiple myeloma, thyroid, non–small cell lung cancers, NHL, and melanoma), primarily osteoblastic (eg, prostate, small cell lung cancer, carcinoid, Hodgkin's lymphoma, medulloblastoma), and malignancies with both osteolytic and osteoblastic components (eg, breast, gastrointestinal and squamous cell carcinomas). Malignant lesions involving the bones can be associated with significant pain and complications such as pathologic fracture, hypercalcemia, and spinal cord compression.

Increased Risk of Malignancies in Certain Autoimmune Rheumatologic Conditions

The increased incidence of malignancies in certain autoimmune rheumatic disorders has long been recognized. Certain long-standing rheumatic syndromes, in particular, rheumatoid arthritis, Felty's syndrome (FS), Sjögren's syndrome, dermatomyositis, systemic sclerosis, systemic lupus erythematosus, and systemic vasculitis, may at times be associated with an increased risk of malignancy. However, tumor markers such as α-fetoprotein, prostate-specific antigen, CA-125, CA 19-9, and CA-3 have low sensitivity and specificity in screening for occult cancer in these patents. On the other hand, the presence of a monoclonal gammopathy in rheumatoid arthritis and the finding of monoclonal antibody 17–9 in Sjögren's syndrome have been described as potential signs of malignant transformation.[6]

Rheumatoid arthritis

The association of malignancies with RA is somewhat controversial. An increased incidence of leukemias and lymphomas in RA has been well recognized since 1978,[10] with the SIR for these cancers estimated to be between 1.9 and 2.7 in different studies.[11] However, colorectal malignancies are consistently reported to have a lower incidence in RA cohorts.[12] This observation has been made across several studies and is thought to be in part caused by the protective effects of the nonsteroidal anti-inflammatory drugs used in the adjunct therapy of these conditions.[13]

T-cell large granular lymphocyte leukemia (T-LGL) may be seen in the setting of chronic inflammation, neutropenia, and RA and is characterized by clonal expansion of cytotoxic T cells. A subset of patients with FS demonstrates polyclonal expansion of LGLs. The polyclonality characteristic of FS help distinguish it from T-LGL, which is associated with monoclonal LGL expansion. Despite this fundamental difference, T-LGL and FS may have clinical similarities. Both follow a chronic inflammatory course and both respond to immunosuppressive therapy.[14] RA can precede or occur concurrently with T-LGL leukemia. The arthritis in this setting can range from mild or intermittent to severe and deforming. Patients with concomitant RA and T-LGL leukemia frequently have antinuclear antibodies and can also occasionally have positive anti-Cyclic Citrullinated Peptide (CCP) antibody and rheumatoid factor.[15]

Systemic lupus erythematosus

An increased incidence of malignancies has also been noted in patients with SLE. The most consistent association exists between SLE and NHLs, which is estimated to be 3 to 4 times higher risk than that in the general population. This association has been shown across several different population cohorts.[16] Additionally, some studies suggest an increased risk of other malignancies, such as lung and hepatobiliary cancers in SLE patients. As an example, a multicenter (23 sites) international cohort of 9547 patients with SLE was observed for a total of 76,948 patient-years, with an average follow-up of 8 years. During the course of the study, 431 cancers occurred. For all cancers combined, the SIR estimate was 1.15 (95% confidence interval [CI], 1.05–1.27). For all hematologic malignancies the SIR was 2.75 (95% CI, 2.13–3.49), and for NHL the SIR was 3.64 (95% CI, 2.63–4.93). The data also suggested an increased risk of lung cancer (SIR, 1.37; 95% CI, 1.05–1.76) and hepatobiliary cancer (SIR, 2.60; 95% CI, 1.25, 4.78).[17]

The same authors published a follow-up article in 2013. This time the study was done in 30 centers and included 16,409 SLE patients. The patients were observed for 121,283 (average 7.4) person-years. In total, 644 cancers occurred. Some cancers, notably hematologic malignancies, were substantially increased (SIR, 3.02; 95% CI, 2.48, 3.63), particularly NHL (SIR, 4.39; 95% CI, 3.46, 5.49) and leukemia. In addition, there was a significant increased risk of cancer of the vulva (SIR, 3.78; 95% CI, 1.52, 7.78) and a modest increased risk of other malignancies such as lung (SIR, 1.30; 95% CI, 1.04, 1.60), thyroid (SIR, 1.76; 95% CI, 1.13, 2.61), and possibly liver (SIR, 1.87; 95% CI, 0.97, 3.27). Interestingly, in this study, decreased risk for breast (SIR, 0.73;

95% CI, 0.61–0.88), endometrial (SIR, 0.44; 95% CI, 0.23–0.77), and possibly ovarian cancers (SIR, 0.64, 95% CI, 0.34–1.10) was observed. The variability of comparative rates across different cancers statistically translates into only a small increased risk across all cancers (SIR, 1.14; 95% CI, 1.05, 1.23). The authors of this study could not draw a conclusion concerning the mechanism of the positive association between SLE and NHL. Similarly, the reason for the observed decreased breast, endometrial, and possibly ovarian cancer risk remains to be elucidated.[18]

Another Swedish study that included 6438 SLE patients noted that the overall 5-year survival rate (50%) and mean age (61 years) for SLE patients with NHL was comparable with those for NHL in the general population. However, the more aggressive NHL subtype of diffuse large B cell lymphoma was reported more frequently in the lupus cohort. This association was independent of history of treatment with cyclophosphamide or azathioprine. Conversely, the NHL risk was higher in patients with hematologic aberrations, sicca symptoms, or pulmonary involvement.[19]

Finally, a recent US population-based cohort study of 133,333 patients with systemic inflammatory disease (SID), which included 58,979 RA patients and 14,513 SLE patients compared the crude incidence rate of high-grade cervical dysplasia and cervical cancer per 100,000 person-years versus a control group of 533,332 patients without SID. They followed up with the patients for 2 years. The risk of high-grade cervical dysplasia and cervical cancer was 1.5 times higher in women with RA and SLE than in those without SID.[20]

Systemic sclerosis and myositis

The most commonly associated malignancy in patients with systemic sclerosis is lung cancer. Smoking is an important risk factor. In an Australian study, scleroderma patients who smoked were 7 times more likely to subsequently develop lung cancer than nonsmokers ($P = .008$). Pulmonary fibrosis and antitopoisomerase antibody did not increase the risk of lung cancer.[21] However, a close temporal relationship between the onset of cancer and scleroderma in patients with antibodies to RNA polymerase I/III has been noted. Malignancy may initiate the scleroderma-specific immune response and drive the disease in a subset of scleroderma patients.[22] The risk of other malignancies, such as esophageal and oropharyngeal malignancies, is also increased.[23] Several scleroderma-like dermatoses, such as scleromyxedema and scleredema, have also been reported in association with paraproteinemia.

Inflammatory myopathies

The association between dermatomyositis and malignancy has been known since 1976, when a review of 258 cases between 1916 to the mid-1970s reported a 5- to 7-fold increase in the incidence of malignancies in patients with dermatomyositis.[24] The risk of underlying malignancy seems to be less impressive with polymyositis and inclusion body myositis. As an example, a study by Buchbinder and colleagues[25] found 116 malignancies in a total of 537 patients with biopsy-proven inflammatory myopathy. The highest risk for malignant disease was associated with dermatomyositis (SIR, 6.2). Cancer risk was also increased in polymyositis but only with SIR of 2.0 and similarly so for inclusion-body myositis (SIR, 2.4). The likelihood of associated cancer diminished with passage of time (SIR, 4.4 in the first year, 3.4 between 1 and 3 years, 2.2 between 3 and 5 years, and 1.6 beyond 5 years [P for trend = .002]).[25] Patients with cancer-associated dermatomyositis have been reported to have more severe cutaneous lesions, dysphagia, and diaphragmatic involvement and to be older.[26]

Vasculitides

The paraneoplastic vasculitides comprise approximately 2% to 5% of all vasculitic syndromes. Leukocytoclastic vasculitis (LCV) accounts for 50% to 60% of paraneoplastic vasculitides and is the most common paraneoplastic vasculitis in both hematologic malignancies and solid tumors.[27] The diagnosis is generally confirmed by skin biopsy, which shows neutrophilic inflammation of vessel walls with endothelial swelling and fibrinoid necrosis in postcapillary venules. Paraneoplastic Henoch-Schönlein purpura (HSP) is a form of LCV and accounts for 15% of paraneoplastic vasculitides. HSP has been reported in association with carcinomas of the lung and urogenital and gastrointestinal tracts. The 2 key patient characteristics of the paraneoplastic forms of HSP are male sex (95%) and older age. In addition, renal involvement is more common in this form of HSP.[28]

Polyarteritis nodosa is a form of vasculitis that accounts for 15% of all paraneoplastic vasculitides and predominantly involves small and medium-sized vessels of the skin, peripheral nervous, and gastrointestinal systems. Hairy cell leukemia is rare and only accounts for 2% of all leukemias. It is arguably the malignancy with the strongest association with paraneoplastic polyarteritis nodosa. One of the possible mechanisms for this association is presumed to be the cross-reactivity of antibodies against hairy cell leukemic cells with vascular endothelial cells.[29]

Paraneoplastic Musculoskeletal Syndromes

Paraneoplastic syndromes are characterized by symptoms that are mediated through hormones and cytokines produced by tumors. Through a variety of cellular or humoral mechanisms these conditions result in clinical manifestations at sites away from the primary tumor or its metastases. Paraneoplastic musculoskeletal syndromes can involve the joints, fasciae, muscles, vessels, or bones. The symptoms generally occur within 2 years of onset of the clinical signs of malignancy, and may be clues for early detection of an occult malignancy. There is a growing list of musculoskeletal syndromes associated with malignancy, which ranges from paraneoplastic synovitis to erythromelalgia. However, a causal relationship between the rheumatologic manifestations and underlying malignancy needs to be established for the symptoms to be considered paraneoplastic. For example, prompt regression of the symptoms after successful treatment of the underlying cancer confirms the association.

Indeed, few syndromes have been found to satisfy the Bradford Hill Criteria for causation.[4] The musculoskeletal syndromes with strongest data supporting their paraneoplastic nature include hypertrophic osteoarthropathy, cancer-associated myositis, paraneoplastic polyarthritis, RS3PE syndrome, palmar fasciitis and polyarthritis (PFPAS), and tumor-induced osteomalacia.

Hypertrophic osteoarthropathy

HOA was first recognized in 1889 by von Bamberger.[30] The clinical association of HOA with underlying lung malignancy was established a few decades later.[31] Patients may present with tibial and femoral bone pain and arthralgia. The physical examination can show soft tissue tenderness in the symptomatic regions, synovitis of the adjacent joints, and clubbing of the digits. Conventional radiographs may show periosteal osseous proliferation. Technetium bone scan further documents increased uptake in the periosteum and involved joints. Acanthosis palmaris (or tripe palms) is a less-recognized finding in patients with HOA and cancer, which presents as hyperkeratosis of the palms with prominence of the dermatoglyphic palmar lines and a gyrated, velvety appearance to the palmar skin.[32] The underlying etiology is thought to be overproduction of several growth factors. One such growth factor is platelet-derived growth factor, which can be released from the small vessels of the fingertips in response to platelet aggregates that have bypassed the lung capillary network in various cardiac and pulmonary diseases. This may cause increased vascularity, permeability, and mesenchymal cell growth that promote new bone formation and clubbing.[33]

Vascular endothelial growth factor (VEGF) is also an important cytokine in the pathogenesis of HOA. Although hypoxemia itself is a strong stimulus for VEGF production, the highest levels of VEGF have been noted in patients with underlying malignancy. VEGF induces vascular hyperplasia, new bone formation, and edema. Removal of the lung tumors results in decreased circulating VEGF levels and at least one reported case of resolution of the skeletal abnormalities.[34] Periostitis and bone pain usually respond well to prostaglandin inhibition by nonsteroidal anti-inflammatory drugs. The refractory cases have been treated with zoledronate in some instances.[35]

Paraneoplastic polyarthritis

Described as an acute onset, RA-like, polyarthritis associated with malignancy, paraneoplastic polyarthritis was first described by Pines and colleagues in 1984.[36] There have since been numerous articles describing this clinical syndrome. The demographics of this condition are different from that of RA, owing to a higher incidence in men (male/female ratio of 1.7:1) and an older median age of onset (approximately 54.2 years). Hematologic or lymphoproliferative malignancies comprise about one-third of the cases. The most frequent solid tumors are adenocarcinomas of the lung and breast, although colon cancer and other solid tumors have also been reported. The arthritis is usually of sudden onset. Patients have significantly elevated C-reactive protein and erythrocyte sedimentation rate. Seropositivity does not rule out the paraneoplastic nature of the arthritis. A total of 27.2% tested positive for rheumatoid factor and 19.0% for antinuclear antibodies.[32] Anticitrullinated protein antibodies can also be present in patients with paraneoplastic arthritis. One case series reported anticitrullinated protein antibody positivity in 7 of 65 patients (10.7%).[37] One of the distinguishing characteristics of this form of arthritis is its lack of response to corticosteroids and other disease-modifying antirheumatic drugs. Typically, the arthritis resolves with adequate treatment of the underlying malignancy. A case series of 26 patients with paraneoplastic arthritis noted that in cases in which the tumor relapsed, 75% of the patients did not experience a relapse of their rheumatic symptoms.[38]

Palmar fasciitis and polyarthritis syndrome

This rare paraneoplastic disorder was first described as shoulder-hand syndrome in 1966 by Bermer.[39] It was not until 1982 when Medsger and colleagues[40] described it as a separate entity in 6 postmenopausal women with malignant ovarian tumors in whom palmar fasciitis and polyarthritis developed. These symptoms preceded the diagnosis of adenocarcinoma of the ovary by 5 to 25 months. All had bilateral pain and limitation of motion of the shoulders and hands and prominent palmar fasciitis and polyarthritis of several other joints. All patients had nonresectable tumors with ascites and peritoneal metastatic seeding. Histologic characteristics included endometrioid carcinoma, poor tumor differentiation, and unusually severe stromal proliferation of fibrous tissue. These patients did not respond to corticosteroids or chemotherapy, and all patients died 2 to 17 months after diagnosis of the neoplasm.[40] A comprehensive review in 2014 described the characteristic features of PFPAS in 100 cases. Most patients had a sudden onset of diffuse painful swelling of both the hands along with marked stiffness. The patients subsequently had nodular thickening of the palmar fascia that was similar to Dupuytren's contracture but much more severe, with loss of function owing to flexion contractures. Similar symptoms were observed in the feet of 20% of patients, reflecting plantar fascia involvement. Some cases had erythematous or acrocyanotic discoloration, but only one satisfied the classic Raynaud's description. Sclerodactyly was absent and capillary microscopy was normal. Some investigators describe advanced cases as possessing "woody hands." Occasionally, the term *groove sign* was used, describing an indentation of the skin over superficial veins when the extremity was raised. The pattern of joint involvement included synovitis of metacarpophalangeal, proximal interphalangeal, and wrists. Adhesive capsulitis of the shoulders was common. Ovarian adenocarcinoma was the most frequent tumor reported (36.8%). Ovarian, breast, and other malignancies of the female reproductive tract comprise 50% of the published cases. Interestingly, inflammatory markers are not particularly elevated, with near-normal erythrocyte sedimentation rate noted in 50% and mild elevation only of C-reactive protein in 70%, of cases.[41] Fibroblast proliferation and increased production of extracellular matrix components are key histologic features of PFPAS. However, the role of soluble stimulators of fibroblast activity, such as transforming growth factor β or connective tissue growth factor, is yet to be proven. A markedly elevated serum soluble interleukin-2 receptor level was noted in one case of gastric carcinoma, suggesting a component of lymphocyte activation in the disease pathogenesis.[42]

Remitting seronegative symmetric synovitis with pitting edema (RS3PE)

RS3PE is characterized by symmetric synovitis of small joints in extremities coupled with significant pitting edema. Patients are usually of advanced age and have negative serology for RA. The condition is briskly responsive to treatment with low-dose corticosteroids. However, a review of the 5 small case series of RS3PE (89 total patients) found malignancy in 22 patients (24.7%) shortly after the onset of symptoms. Five of these cases were of hematopoietic origin. No significant demographic or clinical differences were observed between idiopathic and paraneoplastic cases of RS3PE.[32] VEGF plays a significant role in RS3PE pathogenesis and may explain the synovial hypervascularity and vascular permeability (edema) seen in this condition. Elevated levels of matrix metalloproteinase 3 have been noted in the sera of patients with paraneoplastic form of RS3PE.[43] Both idiopathic and paraneoplastic RS3PE often respond to low-dose prednisone, although the response in the paraneoplastic form can be less dramatic or delayed.[43]

Multicentric reticulohistiocytosis (MRH)

MRH is a rare multisystem granulomatous non–Langerhans cell histiocytosis that presents with severe arthritis and can result in rapid joint destruction. This potentially mutilating arthritis also involves the skin, with dermal infiltration of CD68-positive histiocytes and multinucleated giant cells possessing an eosinophilic ground-glass cytoplasm. These cells form coral-red papular skin lesions (with Köbner's phenomenon) and can also involve the tendon sheath, synovium, bone, and, less commonly liver, salivary glands, kidneys, lymph nodes, heart and lungs.[44] Several other conditions have been reported in association with MRH, including a positive skin tuberculin test (12%–50%), systemic vasculitis, and a variety of underlying internal malignancies (15%–30% of the cases). The malignancies usually occur within 3 years of MRH manifestations and include bronchial, breast, stomach, cervical and liver carcinomas.[45] MRH is relatively resistant to glucocorticoids, methotrexate, and hydroxychloroquine. However, it may respond to tumor necrosis factor α inhibition and to parenteral administration of alendronate.[46]

Erythromelalgia

Erythromelalgia is an uncommon disorder that is defined by the presence of an intense burning pain, increased temperature, and redness of the skin, without evidence of arterial circulatory compromise. The lower extremities are usually involved, and symptoms are worsened by heat and dependency and improve with cooling and elevation of the affected part. The adult form may be idiopathic, but 18% of cases occur in patients with polycythemia vera and essential thrombocythemia. Symptoms of erythromelalgia may precede the development of thrombocytosis by a median of 2.5 years. Interestingly, the disease manifestations in patients with myeloproliferative disorders can sometimes be effectively reversed by a single daily dose of acetylsalicylic acid. The other myeloproliferative disorders associated with erythromelalgia include polycythemia vera, essential thrombocythemia, agnogenic myeloid metaplasia, myelofibrosis, and chronic myelogenous leukemia.[47] In addition, erythromelalgia has been associated with solid organ malignancies such as breast, prostate, ovary, and colon carcinomas as well as thymoma.[48]

Sweet syndrome (acute febrile neutrophilic dermatosis)

Sweet syndrome presents with fever, neutrophilia, arthralgia, and erythematous, tender skin lesions comprising nonvasculitic dermal neutrophilic infiltration. The skin lesions are usually on the face, neck, dorsum of the hands, and upper extremities. The lesions are tender and nonpruritic and can have vesicular and pustular components. The most common underlying malignancies associated with Sweet syndrome are myelogenous leukemia and myelodysplastic syndromes, although association with solid tumors, lymphomas, and plasma cell dyscrasias have also been reported.[49]

Canale-Smith stiff-person or stiff-man syndrome

Canale-Smith stiff-person syndrome (SPS) is a rare condition that presents with progressive muscular rigidity and spasm involving the axial muscles. SPS has been reported in association with several other autoimmune conditions including type I diabetes and thyroiditis, vitiligo, and pernicious anemia. Approximately 35% of SPS patients have type I diabetes.[50]

Glutamic acid decarboxylase (GAD) is an enzyme selectively concentrated in neurons secreting the neurotransmitter γ-aminobutyric acid and in pancreatic β cells. Autoantibodies against GAD have been reported in patients with SPS and concurrent epilepsy and insulin-dependent diabetes mellitus. The presence of this antibody in 20 of 33 patients with SPS has been reported in a previous case series and may be helpful for the diagnosis of this condition.[51] Diabetics have antibodies against a different epitope than the one seen in SPS patients, and their symptoms may start distally and occur in only one limb.

A paraneoplastic SPS has been reported in patients with breast cancer and small cell lung cancers. These patients do not have anti-GAD and anti-islet cell antibodies but may have antibodies against amphiphysin, which is a cytoplasmic protein. Amphiphysin Ab-associated SPS usually occurs in older women with breast cancer and has predilection for involvement of the cervical region. The symptoms respond to benzodiazepines and, at times, corticosteroids treatment. Patients usually experience dramatic improvement after successful treatment of the underlying cancer.[52] Another antibody in patients with SPS is directed against the α1 subunit of the glycine receptor. Patients with this antibody usually do not have cancer but can have progressive encephalomyelitis and myoclonus.[53]

Tumor-induced osteomalacia or oncogenic osteomalacia

This rare paraneoplastic syndrome presents with bone pain, weakness, multiple fractures, height loss, and gait abnormalities. Tumor-induced osteomalacia has been described in association with small mesenchymal tumors that secrete the phosphaturic hormone and fibroblast growth factor 23, with related abnormalities in phosphate and vitamin D metabolism. Laboratory investigations typically show hypophosphatemia caused by renal phosphate wasting, inappropriately normal or low 1,25-dihydroxy vitamin D, and elevated or inappropriately normal plasma fibroblast growth factor 23. In addition, a tumor-induced osteomalacia--like syndrome can also be seen in association with other diseases such as prostate cancer, oat cell cancer, hematologic malignancies, neurofibromatosis, epidermal nevus syndrome, and polyostotic fibrous dysplasia of bone.[54]

Polyneuropathy, organomegaly, endocrinopathy, monoclonal protein, skin changes (POEMS) syndrome

This rare paraneoplastic syndrome is usually secondary to a plasma cell dyscrasia. Patients may also present with papilledema, extravascular volume overload, sclerotic bone lesions, thrombocytosis, and Castleman disease (angiofollicular lymph node hyperplasia). The diagnosis can be confirmed in the presence of elevated blood levels of vascular endothelial growth factor.[55]

Eosinophilic fasciitis

Eosinophilic Fasciitis is characterized by symmetric limb or trunk erythema and edema, followed by the orange peel (peau d'orange) appearance of the skin and subsequent collagenous thickening of the subcutaneous fascia. Eosinophilia is present early in the course of the disease, and the disease spares the skin of the hands and feet. Elevation of an affected limb causes visible indentation along the course of the superficial veins (ie, groove sign). Associated hematologic conditions may include aplastic anemia, myelodysplastic and myeloproliferative disorders, lymphoma, multiple myeloma, and lymphocytic and eosinophilic leukemia.[56]

Lupus-like syndromes

Subacute cutaneous lupus erythematosus (SCLE) is a photosensitive, nonscarring rash that can be seen in association with SLE in 50% of cases; it can also be idiopathic or drug induced. Eighty percent of patients with SCLE have positive results for anti-Ro/SSA antibodies. There are a few reports of SCLE arising in the setting of malignancies such small cell lung cancer.[57] In addition, patients with multiple myeloma and other paraproteinemias can present with positive antinuclear antibodies.

Polymyalgia rheumatica–like syndrome

Polymyalgia rheumatic (PMR) is a disease of older adults who may present with shoulder and hip girdle muscle pain and stiffness. The definitive diagnosis is challenging because of the extensive list of conditions presenting with similar symptoms. A trial of low-dose corticosteroids is commonly met with a prompt and dramatic improvement is the symptoms. A PMR-like paraneoplastic syndrome has been described in association with myelodysplastic diseases and rarely in metastatic cancers. Corticosteroid therapy in these cases does not result in dramatic response. However, successful treatment of the underlying malignancy results in regression of symptoms. When a diagnosis of PMR is established, clues to a potentially fruitful investigation for underlying malignancy include an earlier age of onset, an asymmetric presentation, a sedimentation rate less than 40 or more than 100 mm/h, a poor response to low dose glucocorticoids, and prominent constitutional symptoms.[58]

Pyogenic arthritis

Septic arthritis caused by unusual organisms, such as clostridium septicum[59] and streptococcus bovis,[60] should prompt the search for an occult colon cancer.

SUMMARY

A variety of neoplastic syndromes can present with mucocutaneous and musculoskeletal manifestations and mimic rheumatic conditions. Furthermore, certain autoimmune conditions and associated therapies can result in a higher incidence of particular types of malignancies. Awareness of these associations will result in appropriate screening and more vigilant monitoring of patients at risk.

There is also an expanding array of paraneoplastic conditions that may present as the sole manifestation of an occult malignancy. Therefore, timely recognition of these entities prompt looking for an underlying, otherwise difficult-to-diagnose, malignancy. This would likely result in early diagnosis and appropriate treatment of the associated cancer and better long-term outcome.

It is also critical to suspect an underlying neoplastic condition when certain rheumatologic conditions are unusually refractory to the conventional therapy.

REFERENCES

1. Kankeleit H. Uber primare nichteirige Polymyositis. Dtsch Arch Klin Med 1916; 120:335–49.
2. Zintzaras E, Voulgarelis M, Moutsopoulos HM. The risk of lymphoma development in autoimmune diseases: a meta-analysis. Arch Intern Med 2005;165(20): 2337–44.
3. Naschitz JE. Rheumatic syndromes: clues to occult neoplasia. Curr Opin Rheumatol 2001;13(1):62–6.
4. Hill AB. The environment and disease: association or causation? Proc R Soc Med 1965;58(5):293–300.
5. Villa AR, Kraus A, Alarcon-Segovia D. Autoimmune rheumatic diseases and cancer: evidence of causality?. In: Shoenfeld Y, Gershwin ME, editors. Cancer and autoimmunity. Amsterdam: Elsevier; 2000. p. 111–7.
6. Naschitz JE, Rosner I, Rozenbaum M, et al. Rheumatic syndromes: clues to occult neoplasia. Semin Arthritis Rheum 1999;29(1):43–55.
7. Siegel RL, Miller KD, Jemal A. Cancer statistics, 2016. CA Cancer J Clin 2016; 66(1):7–30.
8. WHO classification of tumours of soft tissue and bone. In: Fletcher CMD, Bridge JA, Hogendoorn PCW, et al, editors. World Health Organization classification of tumours. 4th edition. Lyon (France): International Agency for Research on Cancer; 2013.
9. Garnero P, Buchs N, Zekri J, et al. Markers of bone turnover for the management of patients with bone metastases from prostate cancer. Br J Cancer 2000;82: 858–64.
10. Isomäki H, Hakulinen T, Joutsenlahti U. Excess risk of lymphomas, leukemia and myeloma in patients with rheumatoid arthritis. J Chronic Dis 1978;31:691–6.
11. Chakravarty EF, Genovese MC. Associations between rheumatoid arthritis and malignancy. Rheum Dis Clin North Am 2004;30(2):271–84.
12. Huang WK, Chiou MJ, Kuo CF, et al. No overall increased risk of cancer in patients with rheumatoid arthritis: a nationwide dynamic cohort study in Taiwan. Rheumatol Int 2014;34(10):1379–86.

13. Baron JA. Epidemiology of non-steroidal anti-inflammatory drugs and cancer. Prog Exp Tumor Res 2003;37:1–24.
14. Shah A, Diehl LF, St Clair EW. T cell large granular lymphocyte leukemia associated with rheumatoid arthritis and neutropenia. Clin Immunol 2009;132(2): 145–52.
15. Prochorec-Sobieszek M, Rymkiewicz G, Makuch-Łasica H, et al. Characteristics of T-cell large granular lymphocyte proliferations associated with neutropenia and inflammatory arthropathy. Arthritis Res Ther 2008;10(3):R55.
16. Gayed M, Bernatsky S, Ramsey-Goldman R, et al. Lupus and cancer. Lupus 2009;18(6):479–85.
17. Bernatsky S, Boivin JF, Joseph L, et al. An international cohort study of cancer in systemic lupus erythematosus. Arthritis Rheum 2005;52(5):1481–90.
18. Bernatsky S, Ramsey-Goldman R, Labrecque J, et al. Cancer risk in systemic lupus: an updated international multi-center cohort study. J Autoimmun 2013; 42:130–5.
19. Löfström B, Backlin C, Sundström C, et al. A closer look at non-Hodgkin's lymphoma cases in a national Swedish systemic lupus erythematosus cohort: a nested case-control study. Ann Rheum Dis 2007;66(12):1627–32.
20. Kim SC, Glynn RJ, Giovannucci E, et al. Risk of high-grade cervical dysplasia and cervical cancer in women with systemic inflammatory diseases: a population-based cohort study. Ann Rheum Dis 2015;74:1360–7.
21. Pontifex EK, Hill CL, Roberts-Thomson P. Risk factors for lung cancer in patients with scleroderma: a nested case-control study. Ann Rheum Dis 2007;66:551–3.
22. Shah AA, Rosen A, Hummers L, et al. Close temporal relationship between onset of cancer and scleroderma in patients with RNA polymerase I/III antibodies. Arthritis Rheum 2010;62:2787.
23. Derk CT, Rasheed M, Artlett CM, et al. A cohort study of cancer incidence in systemic sclerosis. J Rheumatol 2006;33:1113–6.
24. Barnes BE, Mawr B. Dermatomyositis and malignancy. A review of the literature. Ann Intern Med 1976;84(1):68–76.
25. Buchbinder R, Forbes A, Hall S, et al. Incidence of malignant disease in biopsy-proven inflammatory myopathy. A population-based cohort study. Ann Intern Med 2001;134(12):1087–95.
26. Ponyi A, Constantin T, Garami M, et al. Cancer-associated myositis: clinical features and prognostic signs. Ann N Y Acad Sci 2005;1051:64–71.
27. Fain O, Hamidou M, Cacoub P, et al. Vasculitides associated with malignancies: analysis of sixty patients. Arthritis Rheum 2007;57(8):1473–80.
28. Park HJ, Ranganathan P. Neoplastic and paraneoplastic vasculitis, vasculopathy, and hypercoagulability. Rheum Dis Clin North Am 2011;37(4):593–606.
29. Hasler P, Kistler P, Gerber H. Vasculitides in hairy cell leukemia. Semin Arthritis Rheum 1995;25(2):134–42.
30. Von Bamberger E. Veränderungen der Röhrenknochen bei Bronchiektasie. Wien Klin Wochenschr 1889;2:226–40 [in German].
31. Craig JW. Hypertrophic pulmonary osteoarthropathy as the first symptom of pulmonary neoplasm. Br Med J 1937;1:750–2.
32. Manger B, Schett G. Paraneoplastic syndromes in rheumatology. Nat Rev Rheumatol 2014;10(11):662–70.
33. Dickinson CJ, Martin JF. Megakaryocytes and platelet clumps as the cause of finger clubbing. Lancet 1987;2:1434–5.

34. Olán F, Portela M, Navarro C, et al. Circulating vascular endothelial growth factor concentrations in a case of pulmonary hypertrophic osteoarthropathy. J Rheumatol 2004;31:614–6.

35. Jayakar BA, Abelson AG, Yao Q. Treatment of hypertrophic osteoarthropathy with zoledronic acid: case report and review of the literature. Semin Arthritis Rheum 2011;41:291–6.

36. Pines A, Kaplinsky N, Olchovsky D, et al. Rheumatoid arthritis-like syndrome: a presenting symptom of malignancy. Report of 3 cases and review of the literature. Eur J Rheumatol Inflamm 1984;7(2):51–5.

37. Kisacik B, Onat AM, Kasifoglu T, et al. Diagnostic dilemma of paraneoplastic arthritis: case series. Int J Rheum Dis 2014;17(6):640–5.

38. Morel J, Deschamps V, Toussirot E, et al. Characteristics and survival of 26 patients with paraneoplastic arthritis. Ann Rheum Dis 2008;67:244–7.

39. Bermer C. Shoulder hand syndrome. A case of unusual etiology. Ann Phys Med 1967;9:168–71.

40. Medsger TA, Dixon JA, Garwood VF. Palmar fasciitis and polyarthritis associated with ovarian carcinoma. Ann Intern Med 1982;96:424–31.

41. Manger B, Schett G. Palmar fasciitis and polyarthritis syndrome—systematic literature review of 100 cases. Semin Arthritis Rheum 2014;44(1):105–11.

42. Enomoto M, Takemura H, Suzuki M, et al. Palmar fasciitis and polyarthritis associated with gastric carcinoma: complete resolution after gastrectomy. Intern Med 2000;39:754–7.

43. Origuchi T, Arima K, Kawashiri SY, et al. High serum matrix metalloproteinase 3 is characteristic of patients with paraneoplastic remitting seronegative symmetrical synovitis with pitting edema syndrome. Mod Rheumatol 2012;22:584–8.

44. Tajirian AL, Malik MK, Robinson-Bostom L, et al. Multicentric reticulohistiocytosis. Clin Dermatol 2006;24:486–92.

45. Hu L, Mei JH, Xia J, et al. Erythema, papules, and arthralgia associated with liver cancer: report of a rare case of multicentric histiocytosis. Int J Clin Exp Pathol 2015;8(3):3304–7.

46. Goto H, Inaba M, Kobayashi K, et al. Successful treatment of multicentric reticulohistiocytosis with alendronate: evidence for a direct effect of bisphosphonate on histiocytes. Arthritis Rheum 2003;48(12):3538.

47. Kurzrock R, Cohen PR. Paraneoplastic erythromelalgia. Clin Dermatol 1993; 11(1):73–82.

48. Han JH, Lee JB, Kim SJ, et al. Paraneoplastic erythromelalgia associated with breast carcinoma. Int J Dermatol 2012;51(7):878–80.

49. Cohen PR, Kurzrock R. Sweet's syndrome revisited: a review of disease concepts. Int J Dermatol 2003;42:761–78.

50. Rakocevic G, Floeter MK. Autoimmune stiff person syndrome and related myelopathies: understanding of electrophysiological and immunological processes. Muscle Nerve 2012;45(5):623–34.

51. Solimena M, Folli F, Aparisi R, et al. Autoantibodies to GABA-ergic neurons and pancreatic beta cells in stiff-man syndrome. N Engl J Med 1990;322(22): 1555–60.

52. Murinson BB, Guarnaccia JB. Stiff-person syndrome with amphiphysin antibodies: distinctive features of a rare disease. Neurology 2008;71(24):1955–8.

53. Hutchinson M, Waters P, McHugh J, et al. Progressive encephalomyelitis, rigidity, and myoclonus: a novel glycine receptor antibody. Neurology 2008;71(16): 1291–2.

54. Chong WH, Molinolo AA, Chen CC, et al. Tumor-induced osteomalacia. Endoc Relat Cancer 2011;18(3):R53–77.
55. Dispenzieri A. POEMS syndrome. Blood Rev 2007;21(6):285–99.
56. Lakhanpal S, Ginsburg WW, Michet CJ, et al. Eosinophilic fasciitis: clinical spectrum and therapeutic response in 52 cases. Semin Arthritis Rheum 1988;17(4): 221–31.
57. Evans KG, Heymann WR. Paraneoplastic subacute cutaneous lupus erythematosus: an under-recognized entity. Cutis 2013;91(1):25–9.
58. Naschitz JE, Slobodin G, Yeshurun D, et al. Atypical polymyalgia rheumatica as a presentation of metastatic cancer. Arch Intern Med 1997;157:2381.
59. Dylewski J, Luterman L. Septic arthritis and Clostridium septicum: a clue to colon cancer. CMAJ 2010;182(13):1446–7.
60. Garcia-Porrua C, Gonzalez-Gay MA, Monterroso JR, et al. Septic arthritis due to Streptococcus bovis as presenting sign of 'silent' colon carcinoma. Rheumatology 2000;39(3):338–9.

Sjögren Syndrome and Other Causes of Sicca in Older Adults

Alan N. Baer, MD[a,b,*], Brian Walitt, MD, MPH[b]

KEYWORDS

- Sjögren syndrome • Dry eye • Aging • Salivary hypofunction • Xerostomia

KEY POINTS

- Symptoms of dry eyes and dry mouth are common in the elderly and most often relate to medication side effects.
- Sjögren syndrome is the prototypic illness that causes dry eyes and dry mouth and is an important diagnostic consideration in older individuals presenting with dry eye and mouth symptoms.
- The diagnosis of Sjögren syndrome requires the presence of anit- Sjögren Syndrome A (SSA) and/or anti-Sjögren syndrome B (SSB) antibodies, or a minor salivary gland biopsy showing at least 1 tightly aggregated periductal lymphocytic aggregate per 4 mm^2 of glandular tissue section (focal lymphocytic sialadenitis with a focus score ≥1).
- Management of Sjögren syndrome requires attention to both the glandular (ocular and oral dryness, glandular enlargement) and extraglandular manifestations (eg, arthritis, pneumonitis, nephritis, vasculitis).

INTRODUCTION

Symptoms of dryness of the eyes, mouth, and vagina (in women) are common among the elderly and have a substantial impact on life quality. The prevalence of these symptoms increases with age and reaches up to 30% in persons more than the age of 65 years, particularly in women.[1–5] Objective evidence of diminished tear or saliva production is much less frequent,[4–6] indicating the weak association between dryness symptoms and objective measures. There are many potential causes for mucosal dryness in the elderly, and multiple factors can contribute in a single individual.

Disclosure: Dr A.N. Baer reports consulting fees from Bristol-Myers Squibb and Novartis.
This article was supported in part by the Intramural Research Program of the NIH, NIDCR.
[a] Division of Rheumatology, Department of Medicine, Johns Hopkins University School of Medicine, 5200 Eastern Avenue, Suite 4000, Mason Lord Center Tower, Baltimore, MD 21224, USA; [b] National Institute of Dental and Craniofacial Research, National Institutes of Health, 10 Center Drive, Bethesda, MD 20892, USA
* Corresponding author. 5200 Eastern Avenue, Suite 4000, Mason Lord Center Tower, Baltimore, MD 21224.
E-mail address: alanbaer@jhmi.edu

Sjögren syndrome (SS) is a chronic systemic autoimmune disease characterized by dry eyes and dry mouth, arising from autoimmune-induced inflammation of the lacrimal and salivary glands. It primarily affects perimenopausal and postmenopausal women and is a prime diagnostic consideration in older patients with mucosal dryness. It can occur in a primary form or in association with another systemic autoimmune disease (termed secondary SS). The reported prevalence of primary SS in population-based studies ranges from 0.01% to 0.09%.[7] SS is present in up to 17% of patients with rheumatoid arthritis,[8,9] a disease whose prevalence reaches 1.1% in the United States.[10] Thus, the overall prevalence is higher, making SS the second most common systemic rheumatic disease.

This article reviews the clinical manifestations, differential diagnosis, and medical evaluation of elderly patients with dry eyes and mouth, as well as the approach to the diagnosis and management of SS.

DRY EYE

Dry eye manifests most often with ocular irritation, including burning, stinging, soreness, and a foreign body sensation. The symptoms are aggravated by exposure to low humidity, wind, or air drafts, as well as prolonged visual attention, including reading. Less frequent symptoms include blurred vision, excess tearing, and blepharospasm.

Dry eye is generally caused by diminished tear production or by excessive tear evaporation[11] (**Box 1**). The former is most often caused by lacrimal gland disease but can result from lacrimal gland duct obstruction or reflex hyposecretion related to corneal sensory loss. Excessive evaporation from meibomian gland dysfunction and other forms of blepharitis is more common. Other causes of dryness include incomplete lid closure during sleep, allergic conjunctivitis, and trachoma.

Tear production and lipid content have been shown to diminish with age[12,13] as a result of changes in lacrimal and meibomian glands, a decreased density of conjunctival goblet cells, and somatosensory nerve impairments.[14] In addition, the elderly frequently have conditions contributing to dry eye, such as the use of medications with anticholinergic side effects, past refractive or cataract surgery,[15] lagophthalmos, blink abnormalities, and conjunctivochalasis.[16]

Box 1
Common causes of dry eye in the elderly

Aqueous Tear Deficiency	Evaporative Tear Deficiency
• SS	• Meibomian gland dysfunction (posterior blepharitis)
• Age-related dry eye	
• Systemic medications (eg, antihistamines, β-blockers, antispasmodics, diuretics)	• Exophthalmos, poor lid apposition, lid deformity
• Lacrimal gland duct obstruction (eg, cicatricial pemphigoid, mucous membrane pemphigoid, trachoma, erythema multiforme, burns)	• Low blink rate
	• Ocular surface disorders (eg, vitamin A deficiency, toxicity from topical drugs/preservatives, contact lens wear)
• Ocular sensory loss leading to reflex hyposecretion (eg, diabetes mellitus, corneal surgery, contact lens wear, trigeminal nerve injury)	• Ocular surface disease (eg, allergic conjunctivitis)
• Lacrimal gland infiltration (eg, sarcoid, lymphoma, graft vs host disease, AIDS, IgG4-related disease)	

Abbreviations: AIDS, acquired immunodeficiency syndrome; Ig, immunoglobulin.

The assessment of dry eye requires multiple tests (**Box 2**). The Schirmer test measures tear production[17] and can be reliably performed by a geriatrician in a clinic setting. A sterile rectangular strip of filter paper, rounded and notched at the proximal end, is folded over the lower eyelid at the midpoint between the middle and lateral fornix of each eye. The patient is then asked to close the eyes gently during the 5-minute duration of the test. The extent of tear wicking or wetting is recorded in millimeters and is normally greater than 5 mm in both eyes. The Schirmer test can be performed with or without anesthesia to measure basal and reflex tear secretion, respectively. This test is imperfect in the elderly, because the results decline with age. In 2 population-based surveys of elderly individuals (65 years or older), the prevalence of an abnormal Schirmer test ranged from 12% to 58%.[2,4]

Ocular surface staining with vital dyes allows slit lamp visualization of devitalized conjunctival cells and corneal epithelial defects. Lissamine green is most commonly used to stain the conjunctiva and fluorescein the cornea. The extent of ocular surface staining is a measure of dryness-induced ocular surface damage, is one of the classification criteria for SS, and can be scored using methods described by van Bijsterveld[18] and by the Sjögren International Collaborative Clinical Alliance (SICCA).[18–20]

The tear breakup time is used to assess the stability of the tear film[21] and is typically abnormal in meibomian gland dysfunction. Tear osmolarity measurement[22,23] is the best for predicting dry eye severity.[23]

XEROSTOMIA AND SALIVARY HYPOFUNCTION

Symptoms of dry mouth, termed xerostomia, include burning, dry lips, alteration of taste, and a sense of having an inadequate amount of saliva. There also may be difficulty speaking, swallowing, and wearing dentures. The need to sip water to swallow dry food is an important marker of reduced salivary function.[24] Halitosis, painful tongue fissures, mucosal ulcers, and pain with ingestion of spicy or acidic foods are common discomforts that may stem from candidal overgrowth on the oral mucosa. The relation between salivation and xerostomia is complex. Dawes[25] showed that healthy patients report dry mouth symptoms when their baseline salivary flow is reduced by 50%, even if the residual salivary flow level remains within the broad range of normal.

Box 2		
Tests used to assess dry eye disease		
Test	**Abnormal Value**	**Significance of Abnormal Test**
Schirmer	<5 mm/5 minute in either eye	Inadequate tear production
Ocular surface staining	Score ≥4 (van Bijsterveld)[18] Score ≥3 (SICCA)[19]	Damage to the ocular surface
Tear break up time	<10 seconds	Poor tear film stability, as seen in meibomian gland dysfunction
Tear osmolarity	≥308 mOsm/L in either eye	Excessive tear evaporation, lacrimal gland disease, or ocular surface inflammation

Abbreviation: SICCA, Sjögren's International Collaborative Clinical Alliance.

Data from van Bijsterveld OP. Diagnostic tests in the sicca syndrome. Arch Ophthalmol 1969;82(1):10–4; and Whitcher JP, Shiboski CH, Shiboski SC, et al. A simplified quantitative method for assessing keratoconjunctivitis sicca from the Sjögren's syndrome International Registry. Am J Ophthalmol 2010;149(3):405–15.

Saliva is produced by the major (parotid, submandibular, sublingual) and myriad submucosal minor salivary glands. The parotid glands only produce saliva on gustatory or olfactory stimulation. Saliva is continually secreted by the sublingual, submandibular, and minor salivary glands. This basal secretion is crucial for maintaining oral health.

Both unstimulated and stimulated salivary flow rates are measured. Saliva that pools in the mouth without stimulation can be collected for 5 to 15 minutes, providing a measure of so-called whole saliva production in a clinic setting (**Box 3**). It is considered the most relevant measure of oral health. Stimulated whole salivary flow rates can be measured with the patient chewing gum or preweighed gauze and are not generally affected by medication use. With special research techniques, stimulated (eg, with lemon juice on the tongue) and unstimulated saliva flow rates can be measured from the individual parotid glands or sublingual/submandibular glands.

Human salivary glands undergo atrophy with age (**Fig. 1**). In morphometric studies, aging was associated with acinar loss and replacement with fat and connective tissue.[26,27] Whole unstimulated saliva flow rates decline with age, which may contribute to the age-dependent increase in dental caries.[28] However, this is not true for stimulated parotid saliva flow rates.[29]

There are multiple potential causes for xerostomia and salivary hypofunction in the elderly (**Box 4**).[6] Side effects from medications commonly used in the geriatric population are the most common.

VAGINAL DRYNESS

Vaginal dryness, dyspareunia, and vulvar pruritus are common symptoms among postmenopausal women. These symptoms relate to menopause-related decreases in the levels of estrogen and other sex steroids but can also have other causes. In 2014, 2 international societies recommended that the range of symptoms and signs associated with menopause be termed the genitourinary syndrome of menopause.[30] These symptoms include genital dryness, burning, irritation, inadequate lubrication, dyspareunia, urinary urgency, dysuria, and recurrent urinary tract infections. Similar symptoms are also seen with infectious vaginitis, irritant or allergic vulvitis or vaginitis,

---

Box 3
Measurement of unstimulated whole salivary flow rate

Unstimulated whole saliva collection measures saliva production under resting or basal conditions. The patient should not have had anything to eat or drink for 90 minutes before the procedure. The use of a parasympathomimetic should be discontinued for 12 hours before the procedure, and the use of artificial saliva should be stopped 3 hours before. During the collection procedure, the patient is instructed to minimize actions that can stimulate saliva (talking, increased orofacial movement) and should not swallow. At time 0, any saliva present in the mouth is cleared by swallowing. For the subsequent 5 minutes, any saliva collected in the mouth is emptied into a preweighed tube every minute (ie, 5 times). This collecting tube then is weighed to determine a postcollection weight. The difference between the precollection and postcollection weight is determined, and this represents the unstimulated whole saliva production for 5 minutes. To convert to a volume of saliva from the weight of saliva, an assumption is made that saliva is similar to water, with 1 g of water/saliva at 4°C equaling 1 mL of saliva/water.

Less than 0.100 mL/min is considered a reduced unstimulated salivary flow rate.

From Wu AJ. Optimizing dry mouth treatment for individuals with Sjögren's syndrome. Rheum Dis Clin North Am 2008;34(4):1004; with permission.

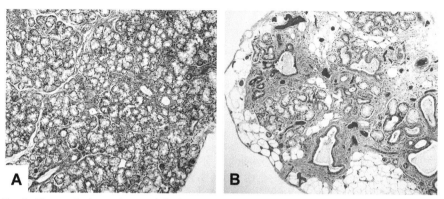

Fig. 1. Histopathology of minor labial salivary glands. The sections are from biopsies of a 28-year-old woman (*A*) and a 65-year-old woman (*B*), shown at the same magnification. Neither had Sjögren syndrome. (*A*) This histopathologic section shows normal tissue, with confluent mucous acini and normal-sized intralobular ducts. (*B*) In contrast, this section shows extensive acinar loss, interstitial fibrosis, ductal dilatation, and fatty replacement. These changes are often seen to varying degrees in older patients (H&E stain, original magnification ×100).

vulvovaginal dermatoses, hypertonic pelvic floor muscle dysfunction, painful bladder syndrome/interstitial cystitis, vulvodynia, and pudendal neuralgia.[30]

In women affected by SS, vaginal dryness can be severe and affect sexual ability and pleasure.[31] There is scant information regarding the cause of this dryness. One hypothesis is that the Skene and related glands of the vaginal introitus are affected in the same manner as exocrine glands found elsewhere.[32] There has been no histopathologic confirmation of this to date.

SJÖGREN SYNDROME

SS is the prototypic illness of dryness of the eyes and mouth. It is a systemic autoimmune disease characterized by lymphocytic infiltration of the salivary and lacrimal glands. This chronic inflammatory process gradually leads to glandular injury and related dysfunction over the course of years, eventually causing the cardinal symptoms of dry eyes and mouth. Keratoconjunctivitis sicca is the term coined by Henrik Sjögren[33] in 1933 to describe the dry eye component of this syndrome. Key features are shown in **Box 5**.

SS disease onset is uncommon after the age of 65 or 70 years.[40,41] Older patients with SS, compared with younger ones, have a lower frequency of serologic abnormalities,

---

Box 4
Common causes of dry mouth in the elderly

- Medications, including antidepressants, anticholinergics, antispasmodics, antihypertensives, antihistamines, sedatives, and diuretics
- SS
- Diabetes mellitus
- Head and neck irradiation
- Dehydration
- Parkinson disease

Box 5
Key clinical features of Sjögren syndrome

- Predominant involvement of women, with female to male ratios more than 10:1.
- Diagnosis most commonly established in the fifth and sixth decades of life, although symptoms of dryness may precede the diagnosis by many years.
- Affects individuals across the age spectrum, including children, but most commonly women in the perimenopausal years of life.
- Extraglandular manifestations in approximately 50% of patients, including constitutional symptoms (eg, fatigue and mild cognitive impairment) and other systemic manifestations, with involvement of diverse organ systems.
- Presence of anti-SSA/Ro and anti-SSB/La in 60% to 80% of patients.[34–37]
- Increased risk of B-cell non-Hodgkin lymphoma, particularly MALT and diffuse B-cell lymphoma. The relative risk of non-Hodgkin lymphoma ranges from 4.8 for primary to 9.6 for secondary SS,[38] with an estimated lifetime risk of 5% to 10%.[39]

Abbreviation: MALT, mucosa-associated lymphoid tissue.
  Data from Refs.[34–39]

---

such as anti-SSA, anti-SSB, rheumatoid factor, and hyperglobulinemia.[42] Parotid enlargement, arthralgia, and Raynaud phenomenon are also less common, although higher frequencies of lung involvement and anemia have been noted.[41] A distinct subset of older patients with SS with anticentromere antibodies is characterized by Raynaud phenomenon, overlap features of limited systemic sclerosis, and more severe salivary and lacrimal gland dysfunction.[43]

The clinical presentation of SS is varied, but is most often that of mucosal dryness (**Box 6**).

SS is associated with a variety of systemic manifestations (**Box 7**). Some are direct manifestations of the disease, whereas others represent coincidental autoimmune diseases. Apart from symptoms of fatigue, joint pain, and mild cognitive impairment (often termed brain fog), the prevalence of these organ-specific manifestations is each less than 20%.[44]

The natural history is generally one of stability, with a slow decline in lacrimal and salivary gland function. It is not characterized by the types of disease flares seen in systemic lupus or rheumatoid arthritis, but patients may report periods of worsening sicca or fatigue. There is no increase in overall mortality according to a recent

---

Box 6
Modes of presentation of Sjögren syndrome

- Symptoms or signs of dry eyes and mouth
- Episodic or persistent salivary gland enlargement
- Sudden increase in dental caries
- An established connective tissue disease complicated by dry eyes or mouth
- Extraglandular disease (eg, annular erythema, cryoglobulinemia, peripheral neuropathy, or interstitial pneumonitis)
- Abnormal serologic test, such as anti-SSA and/or anti-SSB antibodies
- MALT lymphoma of a salivary gland

Box 7	
Systemic manifestations of Sjögren syndrome	
Organ Involvement	**Manifestation**
Constitutional	Fatigue
	Mild cognitive disturbance
Musculoskeletal	Arthritis/arthralgia
	Myositis (especially inclusion body myositis)
Cutaneous	Annular erythema
	Xerosis
	Palpable purpura
Pulmonary	Interstitial pneumonitis
	Follicular bronchiolitis
Vascular	Raynaud
	Vasculitis
Gastrointestinal	Atrophic gastritis
	Primary biliary cirrhosis
Endocrine	Autoimmune thyroid disease
Cardiac	Pericarditis
Renal	Interstitial nephritis with renal tubular acidosis
	Membranoproliferative glomerulonephritis
Hematologic	Leukopenia, neutropenia
	Thrombocytopenia
	Anemia
	Monoclonal gammopathy
	Cryoglobulinemia
Lymphoproliferative	Lymphoma
Neurologic	Peripheral neuropathy
	Ataxic ganglionopathy
	Myelitis (including neuromyelitis optica)

meta-analysis, but patients with specific extraglandular manifestations, including those with vasculitis, cryoglobulinemia, pulmonary disease, and lymphoma, have been identified as having higher mortalities.[45,46]

DIAGNOSIS OF SJÖGREN SYNDROME

The diagnosis requires evidence of autoimmune-induced inflammation targeting the salivary or lacrimal glands. Two sets of classification criteria are currently in use: the 2002 American-European Criteria Group (**Box 8**) and the 2012 American College of Rheumatology provisional classification criteria (**Box 9**).[47,48] Both require that the patient have either anti-SSA and/or anti-SSB antibodies or a minor salivary gland biopsy showing focal lymphocytic sialadenitis with a focus score greater than or equal to 1. These 2 sets of criteria have good concordance.[49] However, both criteria sets have limitations, and thus a new set of international consensus criteria is in development. The authors use these current classification criteria as a general guide, and establish the diagnosis if a patient has an objective measure of ocular and/or oral dryness or characteristic imaging abnormalities (eg, by ultrasonography, magnetic resonance [MR], or computed tomography [CT]), coupled with anti-SSA antibodies or a positive lip biopsy.

For practicing geriatricians, the authors recommend that patients suspected of having SS be evaluated as follows:

- History, seeking a history of persistent symptoms of dry eyes and/or mouth. Validated screening questions are included in the American-European Classification Criteria (see **Box 8**)

Box 8
American-European Consensus Group Revised International Classification Criteria for Sjögren syndrome

1. Ocular symptoms: a positive response to at least 1 of the following questions:
   a. Have you had daily, persistent, troublesome dry eyes for more than 3 months?
   b. Do you have a recurrent sensation of sand or gravel in the eyes?
   c. Do you use tear substitutes more than 3 times a day?

2. Oral symptoms: a positive response to at least 1 of the following questions:
   a. Have you had a daily feeling of dry mouth for more than 3 months?
   b. Have you had recurrently or persistently swollen salivary glands as an adult?
   c. Do you frequently drink liquids to aid in swallowing dry food?

3. Ocular signs: objective evidence of ocular involvement, defined as a positive result for at least 1 of the following 2 tests:
   a. Schirmer test, performed without anesthesia (<5 mm in 5 min)
   b. Rose Bengal score or other ocular dye score (>4 according to van Bijsterveld scoring system)

4. Histopathology: in minor salivary glands (obtained through normal-appearing mucosa) focal lymphocytic sialoadenitis, evaluated by an expert histopathologist, with a focus score greater than 1, defined as several lymphocytic foci (which are adjacent to normal-appearing mucous acini and contain more than 50 lymphocytes) per 4 mm^2 of glandular tissue.

5. Salivary gland involvement: objective evidence of salivary gland involvement defined by a positive result for at least 1 of the following diagnostic tests:
   a. Unstimulated whole salivary flow (<1.5 mL in 15 min)
   b. Parotid sialography showing the presence of diffuse sialectasias (punctate, cavitary, or destructive pattern), without evidence of obstruction in the major ducts
   c. Salivary scintigraphy showing delayed uptake, reduced concentration, and/or delayed excretion of tracer

6. Autoantibodies: presence in the serum of the following autoantibodies:
   a. Antibodies to Ro(SSA) or La(SSB) antigens, or both

For primary SS

In patients without any potentially associated disease, primary SS may be defined as follows:
a. The presence of any 4 of the 6 items indicates primary SS, as long as either item IV (histopathology) or VI (serology) is positive
b. The presence of any 3 of the 4 objective criteria items (ie, items III, IV, V, VI)
c. The classification tree procedure represents a valid alternative method for classification, although it should be more properly used in clinical-epidemiologic survey

For secondary SS

In patients with a potentially associated disease (eg, another well-defined connective tissue disease), the presence of item I or item II plus any 2 from among items III, IV, and V may be considered to indicate secondary SS

Exclusion criteria: past head and neck radiation treatment; hepatitis C infection; acquired immunodeficiency disease (eg, AIDS); preexisting lymphoma; sarcoidosis; graft-versus-host disease; use of anticholinergic drugs (since a time shorter than 4-fold the half-life of the drug)

From Vitali C, Bombardieri S, Jonsson R, et al. Classification criteria for Sjögren's syndrome: a revised version of the European criteria proposed by the American-European Consensus Group. Ann Rheum Dis 2002;61(6):557; with permission.

Box 9
American College of Rheumatology provisional criteria for classification of Sjögren syndrome

The classification of SS, which applies to individuals with signs/symptoms that may be suggestive of SS, is met in patients who have at least 2 of the following 3 objective features:
1. Positive serum anti-SSA/Ro and/or anti-SSB/La or (positive rheumatoid factor and antinuclear antibody (ANA) titer greater than or equal to 1:320)
2. Labial salivary gland biopsy showing focal lymphocytic sialadenitis with a focus score greater than or equal to 1 focus/4 mm^2
3. Keratoconjunctivitis sicca with ocular staining score greater than or equal to 3 (assuming that individual is not currently using daily eye drops for glaucoma and has not had corneal surgery or cosmetic eyelid surgery in the last 5 years)

Prior diagnosis of any of the following conditions excludes participation in SS studies or therapeutic trials because of overlapping clinical features or interference with criteria tests:
• History of head and neck radiation treatment
• Hepatitis C infection
• AIDS
• Sarcoidosis
• Amyloidosis
• Graft-versus-host disease
• IgG4-related disease

From Shiboski SC, Shiboski CH, Criswell L, et al. American College of Rheumatology classification criteria for Sjögren's syndrome: a data-driven, expert consensus approach in the Sjögren's International Collaborative Clinical Alliance cohort. Arthritis Care Res (Hoboken) 2012;64(4):484; with permission.

• Examination, seeking signs of salivary hypofunction and of a systemic rheumatic disease
  ○ Oral examination
    ■ Is there enlargement of the lacrimal or major salivary glands? What is the texture of the major salivary glands? Are there discrete nodules or masses?
    ■ Does saliva pool under the elevated tongue when observed over the course of 1 minute?
    ■ Does the tongue have deep fissures, a hyperlobulated appearance, or absence of filiform papillae on its surface?
  ○ General examination
    ■ Look for sclerodactyly, palpable purpura, synovitis, basilar pulmonary rales
• Laboratory testing
  ○ Screen for ANA (tested by immunofluorescence assay), anti-SSA (Ro), and anti-SSB (La), and rheumatoid factor. Anti-SSA and anti-SSB antibodies can be present despite a negative ANA test.
  ○ A complete blood count, urinalysis, and chemistry profile may reveal abnormalities supportive of SS, including leukopenia and neutropenia, hyperglobulinemia, renal impairment, and proteinuria.
• Ophthalmologic examination
  ○ Schirmer testing is an appropriate initial test. A formal ophthalmologic examination serves not only to confirm the diagnosis of dry eye but also to define the contributing causes, such as meibomian gland dysfunction and conjunctivochalasis. Guidelines for this evaluation can be found at https://sicca-online.ucsf.edu/documents/eye-exam-SOP.pdf
• Sialometry
  ○ Documentation of salivary hypofunction is only necessary if the eye examination does not show dry eye disease (see **Box 3**).

- Labial gland biopsy
  - A labial gland biopsy, best performed by an oral surgeon, is required for diagnosis if the patient lacks anti-SSA and/or anti-SSB antibodies. The biopsy also has value in excluding alternative diagnoses (eg, sarcoid, amyloid, mucosa-associated lymphoid tissue lymphoma, and immunoglobulin [Ig] G4–related disease). Guidelines for its performance can be found at https://sicca-online. ucsf.edu/documents/Oral-Saliva-SOP.pdf.
- Imaging (**Fig. 2**)
  - Salivary gland ultrasonography is favored because of its low cost and lack of ionizing radiation. The presence of multiple ovoid hypoechoic lesions, often bounded by hyperechoic bands, correlates with markers of more severe disease. These imaging abnormalities have high specificity for the diagnosis, but only moderate sensitivity.[50–54]

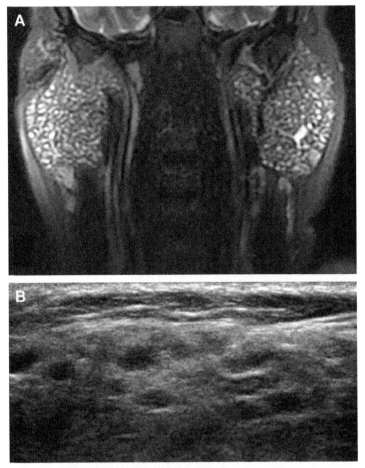

Fig. 2. Imaging techniques in Sjögren syndrome. This patient has bilateral symmetric parotid gland enlargement, seen best on the T2 fat-suppressed MR images (*A*). Note the multiple T2-hyperintense foci scattered throughout both glands, a characteristic finding. With ultrasonography (*B*), multiple hypoechoic rounded lesions with convex borders are noted throughout the glandular parenchyma. In normal parotid gland tissue, the parenchyma has a homogeneous appearance with ultrasonography.

○ CT imaging is not recommended because of the radiation exposure. However, the presence of multiple punctate calcifications within the parotid glands has high specificity.[55]

○ MRI of the parotid glands may reveal heterogeneity of signal intensity on both T1-weighted and T2-weighted images, with both hypointense and hyperintense foci measuring 1 to 4 mm in diameter.[56]

Be aware of certain common pitfalls in the diagnostic evaluation. Antibodies to SSA and SSB are not specific. They are found in systemic lupus and inflammatory myopathies and are seen in up to 0.9% of healthy women in the US population.[57] Labial gland biopsies of older adults are also subject to misinterpretation. The histopathology of the minor salivary gland, termed focal lymphocytic sialadenitis, is characterized by lymphocytic aggregates that surround intralobular salivary ducts (**Fig. 3**) and are adjacent to normal-appearing mucus-secreting acini. The number of these lymphocytic aggregates per 4 mm^2 of glandular tissue section equates to the focus score. A score greater than or equal to 1 is a criterion for the classification of SS and has been validated as the best cut-off value differentiating SS from non-SS controls.[58] Because chronic inflammation of the salivary gland can also arise from ductal obstruction and other forms of glandular injury, care must be taken to exclude from the focus score lymphocytic aggregates in areas of severe acinar loss, ductal dilatation, and fibrosis (**Fig. 4**).

In elderly patients, the differential diagnosis of SS primarily includes alternative causes of sicca symptoms, salivary and/or lacrimal gland enlargement, and the characteristic serologic abnormalities.

- Sicca complex in the elderly: age-related interstitial fibrosis, acinar atrophy, and nonspecific chronic inflammation in the labial gland biopsy may be misinterpreted as indicating SS (see **Fig. 4**).
- Salivary and/or lacrimal gland enlargement: in elderly patients, particular attention should be paid to the possibility of lymphoma. IgG-4 related disease is most common in elderly men. It may present as unilateral submandibular gland enlargement (Küttner tumor) or parotid and lacrimal gland enlargement. Other diagnostic possibilities include amyloid infiltration, sarcoidosis, human immunodeficiency virus infection, bulimia, and hyperlipoproteinemia.

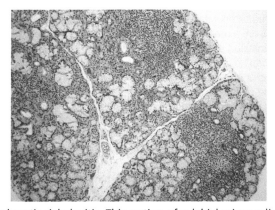

Fig. 3. Focal lymphocytic sialadenitis. This section of a labial minor salivary gland biopsy shows the typical features of focal lymphocytic sialadenitis. Note the tightly aggregated lymphocytes surrounding ducts and adjacent to normal-appearing mucous acini. At least 3 foci are evident (H&E stain, original magnification ×100).

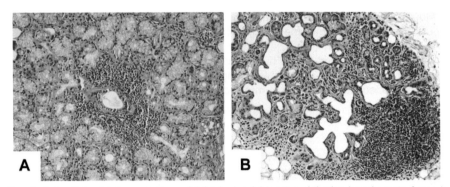

Fig. 4. Potential misinterpretation of labial gland biopsies. (*A*) The lymphocytic focus is typical of that seen in focal lymphocytic sialadenitis, being centered on a duct and adjacent to normal-appearing mucus-secreting acini. (*B*) In contrast, the lymphocytic focus here is present within a gland lobule marked by interstitial fibrosis, ductal dilatation, and marked acinar loss. This focus should not be interpreted as representative of Sjögren syndrome (H&E stain, original magnification ×100).

- Serologic abnormalities: antinuclear antibodies, rheumatoid factor, and monoclonal proteins are more prevalent in the elderly population.[57] Thus, positive tests must be interpreted cautiously when they coincide with symptoms or signs of oral or ocular dryness.

MANAGEMENT OF SJÖGREN SYNDROME

Most patients only require topical and systemic treatments directed at alleviating their ocular, oral, and vaginal dryness; preventing dental decay; and managing oral candidiasis. Patients with systemic manifestations, including those with joint pain, skin lesions, and internal organ involvement, may benefit from immunomodulatory treatments. All patients with SS require monitoring for disease complications, especially lymphoma.

Management of ocular dryness depends on its severity and the patient's response to therapy.[59] Avoidance of wind and smoke, and the use of protective eyewear, can be helpful for all patients. Artificial tears with a demulcent (eg, methylcellulose, propylene glycol, and glycerin) are a mainstay of treatment. Patients should use preservative-free drops if drops are instilled 4 or more times a day. Use of thicker ocular gels and ointments before bed can help with dryness that occurs during sleep. Supplementation of the diet with omega-3 essential fatty acids has been shown to be of benefit. Use of topical cyclosporine and steroid solutions can be useful in a variety of dry eye conditions but should be undertaken in consultation with an ophthalmologist. Punctal plugs to preserve tears are often used in moderate to severe dry eye. Patients with more severe dry eye disease may require the use of moisture chamber spectacles, autologous serum tears, contact lenses, or scleral prostheses.

Prevention of oral dryness includes maintaining good hydration and avoiding medications that worsen dryness. Patients should be counseled to be more aware of factors that can aggravate dryness, such as low-humidity environments and mouth breathing. Frequent sips of oral solutions can be helpful, with options ranging from water to artificial saliva. Sucking on sugar-free hard candies helps stimulate saliva flow. Oral hygiene and dental care are essential in preserving dentition in persons with pathologic oral dryness.

Muscarinic agonists, such as pilocarpine and cevimeline, can substantially increase saliva and, to a lesser extent, tear flow. However, overall tolerance of these agents may be hampered by cholinergic side effects of excessive sweating, increased urinary frequency, flushing, chills, rhinitis, nausea, and diarrhea. Care must be taken when these medications are prescribed to the elderly.

Vaginal moisturizers and lubricants, including olive and vitamin E oils, are initial treatment options for vaginal dryness. Vitamin E capsules can be opened and the oil used in and around the vagina. A suppository containing hyaluronic acid, vitamin E, and vitamin A, used once daily for 14 days, then once every other day for the next 2 weeks, can be effective.[60] Obtaining these suppositories requires a compounding pharmacist. Topical estrogen cream may help if symptoms do not improve with these other measures.

Hydroxychloroquine is commonly used for the management of joint pain and/or fatigue. However, clinical trials with this drug have shown mixed results, with none showing major clinical improvements.[61–63] The effect of immunosuppressive therapies on the glandular manifestations has been disappointing to date. The effect of rituximab on SS dryness is still being evaluated, with potential benefit being observed in a small, double-blind, placebo-controlled trial[64] but not in a larger one.[65] Prolonged therapy may be required for benefit.[66]

SUMMARY

Dryness of the eyes and mouth is a prevalent symptom among the elderly, most often related to the side effects of medications. However, there is a broad differential diagnosis for each symptom, and careful evaluation is important to define the cause and correct treatment. SS is the prototypic disease that leads to these symptoms and primarily affects perimenopausal women. The diagnosis requires demonstration of an autoimmune disease underlying the sicca manifestations, either serologically or pathologically. Management can involve both topical and systemic therapies.

REFERENCES

1. Johansson AK, Johansson A, Unell L, et al. Self-reported dry mouth in Swedish population samples aged 50, 65 and 75 years. Gerodontology 2012;29(2): e107–15.
2. Lin PY, Tsai SY, Cheng CY, et al. Prevalence of dry eye among an elderly Chinese population in Taiwan: the Shihpai Eye Study. Ophthalmology 2003;110(6): 1096–101.
3. Billings RJ, Proskin HM, Moss ME. Xerostomia and associated factors in a community-dwelling adult population. Community Dent Oral Epidemiol 1996; 24(5):312–6.
4. Schein OD, Munoz B, Tielsch JM, et al. Prevalence of dry eye among the elderly. Am J Ophthalmol 1997;124(6):723–8.
5. Hay EM, Thomas E, Pal B, et al. Weak association between subjective symptoms or and objective testing for dry eyes and dry mouth: results from a population based study. Ann Rheum Dis 1998;57(1):20–4.
6. Liu B, Dion MR, Jurasic MM, et al. Xerostomia and salivary hypofunction in vulnerable elders: prevalence and etiology. Oral Surg Oral Med Oral Pathol Oral Radiol 2012;114(1):52–60.
7. Qin B, Wang J, Yang Z, et al. Epidemiology of primary Sjögren's syndrome: a systematic review and meta-analysis. Ann Rheum Dis 2015;74(11):1983–9.

8. Uhlig T, Kvien TK, Jensen JL, et al. Sicca symptoms, saliva and tear production, and disease variables in 636 patients with rheumatoid arthritis. Ann Rheum Dis 1999;58(7):415–22.

9. Carmona L, Gonzalez-Alvaro I, Balsa A, et al. Rheumatoid arthritis in Spain: occurrence of extra-articular manifestations and estimates of disease severity. Ann Rheum Dis 2003;62(9):897–900.

10. Gabriel SE, Crowson CS, O'Fallon WM. The epidemiology of rheumatoid arthritis in Rochester, Minnesota, 1955-1985. Arthritis Rheum 1999;42(3):415–20.

11. The definition and classification of dry eye disease: report of the Definition and Classification Subcommittee of the International Dry Eye WorkShop (2007). Ocul Surf 2007;5(2):75–92.

12. Henderson JW, Prough WA. Influence of age and sex on flow of tears. Arch Ophthalmol 1950;43(2):224–31.

13. Mathers WD, Lane JA, Zimmerman MB. Tear film changes associated with normal aging. Cornea 1996;15(3):229–34.

14. Gipson IK. Age-related changes and diseases of the ocular surface and cornea. Invest Ophthalmol Vis Sci 2013;54(14):ORSF48–53.

15. Kasetsuwan N, Satitpitakul V, Changul T, et al. Incidence and pattern of dry eye after cataract surgery. PLoS One 2013;8(11):e78657.

16. Chhadva P, Alexander A, McClellan AL, et al. The impact of conjunctivochalasis on dry eye symptoms and signs. Invest Ophthalmol Vis Sci 2015;56(5):2867–71.

17. Cho P, Yap M. Schirmer test. I. A review. Optom Vis Sci 1993;70(2):152–6.

18. van Bijsterveld OP. Diagnostic tests in the sicca syndrome. Arch Ophthalmol 1969;82(1):10–4.

19. Whitcher JP, Shiboski CH, Shiboski SC, et al. A simplified quantitative method for assessing keratoconjunctivitis sicca from the Sjögren's Syndrome International Registry. Am J Ophthalmol 2010;149(3):405–15.

20. Bron AJ, Evans VE, Smith JA. Grading of corneal and conjunctival staining in the context of other dry eye tests. Cornea 2003;22(7):640–50.

21. Sweeney DF, Millar TJ, Raju SR. Tear film stability: a review. Exp Eye Res 2013; 117:28–38.

22. Lemp MA, Bron AJ, Baudouin C, et al. Tear osmolarity in the diagnosis and management of dry eye disease. Am J Ophthalmol 2011;151(5):792–8.e1.

23. Potvin R, Makari S, Rapuano CJ. Tear film osmolarity and dry eye disease: a review of the literature. Clin Ophthalmol 2015;9:2039–47.

24. Fox PC, Busch KA, Baum BJ. Subjective reports of xerostomia and objective measures of salivary gland performance. J Am Dent Assoc 1987;115(4): 581–4.

25. Dawes C. Physiological factors affecting salivary flow rate, oral sugar clearance, and the sensation of dry mouth in man. J Dent Res 1987;66(Spec No):648–53.

26. Scott J, Flower EA, Burns J. A quantitative study of histological changes in the human parotid gland occurring with adult age. J Oral Pathol 1987;16(10):505–10.

27. Syrjanen S. Age-related changes in structure of labial minor salivary glands. Age Ageing 1984;13(3):159–65.

28. Percival RS, Challacombe SJ, Marsh PD. Flow rates of resting whole and stimulated parotid saliva in relation to age and gender. J Dent Res 1994;73(8): 1416–20.

29. Ship JA, Pillemer SR, Baum BJ. Xerostomia and the geriatric patient. J Am Geriatr Soc 2002;50(3):535–43.

30. Portman DJ, Gass ML. Vulvovaginal atrophy terminology consensus conference panel. Genitourinary syndrome of menopause: new terminology for vulvovaginal

atrophy from the International Society for the Study of Women's Sexual Health and the North American Menopause Society. Menopause 2014;21(10):1063–8.

31. Maddali Bongi S, Del Rosso A, Orlandi M, et al. Gynaecological symptoms and sexual disability in women with primary Sjögren's syndrome and sicca syndrome. Clin Exp Rheumatol 2013;31(5):683–90.

32. Bloch KJ, Buchanan WW, Wohl MJ, et al. Sjögren's syndrome. A clinical, pathological, and serological study of sixty-two cases. Medicine (Baltimore) 1965;44: 187–231.

33. Sjögren H. Zur Kenntnis der Keratoconjunctivitis sicca (Keratitis filiformis bei Hypofunktion der Tränendrüsen). Acta Ophthalmol (Copenh) 1933;11(Suppl 2): 1–151.

34. Malladi AS, Sack KE, Shiboski SC, et al. Primary Sjögren's syndrome as a systemic disease: a study of participants enrolled in an international Sjögren's syndrome registry. Arthritis Care Res (Hoboken) 2012;64(6):911–8.

35. Theander E, Henriksson G, Ljungberg O, et al. Lymphoma and other malignancies in primary Sjögren's syndrome: a cohort study on cancer incidence and lymphoma predictors. Ann Rheum Dis 2006;65(6):796–803.

36. Lin DF, Yan SM, Zhao Y, et al. Clinical and prognostic characteristics of 573 cases of primary Sjögren's syndrome. Chin Med J (Engl) 2010;123(22):3252–7.

37. Ramos-Casals M, Brito-Zeron P, Perez-De-Lis M, et al. Sjögren syndrome or Sjögren disease? The histological and immunological bias caused by the 2002 criteria. Clin Rev Allergy Immunol 2010;38(2–3):178–85.

38. Ekstrom Smedby K, Vajdic CM, Falster M, et al. Autoimmune disorders and risk of non-Hodgkin lymphoma subtypes: a pooled analysis within the InterLymph Consortium. Blood 2008;111(8):4029–38.

39. Papageorgiou A, Ziogas DC, Mavragani CP, et al. Predicting the outcome of Sjögren's syndrome-associated non-Hodgkin's lymphoma patients. PLoS One 2015; 10(2):e0116189.

40. Botsios C, Furlan A, Ostuni P, et al. Elderly onset of primary Sjögren's syndrome: clinical manifestations, serological features and oral/ocular diagnostic tests. Comparison with adult and young onset of the disease in a cohort of 336 Italian patients. Joint Bone Spine 2011;78(2):171–4.

41. Ramos-Casals M, Solans R, Rosas J, et al. Primary Sjögren syndrome in Spain: clinical and immunologic expression in 1010 patients. Medicine (Baltimore) 2008;87(4):210–9.

42. Haga HJ, Jonsson R. The influence of age on disease manifestations and serological characteristics in primary Sjögren's syndrome. Scand J Rheumatol 1999;28(4):227–32.

43. Baer AN, Medrano L, McAdams-DeMarco M, et al. Anti-centromere antibodies are associated with more severe exocrine glandular dysfunction in Sjögren's syndrome: analysis of the Sjögren's International Collaborative Clinical Alliance cohort. Arthritis Care Res (Hoboken) 2016. [Epub ahead of print].

44. Brito-Zeron P, Ramos-Casals M, EULAR-SS Task Force Group. Advances in the understanding and treatment of systemic complications in Sjögren's syndrome. Curr Opin Rheumatol 2014;26(5):520–7.

45. Singh AG, Singh S, Matteson EL. Rate, risk factors and causes of mortality in patients with Sjögren's syndrome: a systematic review and meta-analysis of cohort studies. Rheumatology (Oxford) 2016;55(3):450–60.

46. Nannini C, Jebakumar AJ, Crowson CS, et al. Primary Sjögren's syndrome 1976-2005 and associated interstitial lung disease: a population-based study of incidence and mortality. BMJ Open 2013;3(11):e003569.

47. Vitali C, Bombardieri S, Jonsson R, et al. Classification criteria for Sjögren's syndrome: a revised version of the European criteria proposed by the American-European Consensus Group. Ann Rheum Dis 2002;61(6):554–8.
48. Shiboski SC, Shiboski CH, Criswell L, et al. American College of Rheumatology classification criteria for Sjögren's syndrome: a data-driven, expert consensus approach in the Sjögren's International Collaborative Clinical Alliance cohort. Arthritis Care Res (Hoboken) 2012;64(4):475–87.
49. Rasmussen A, Ice JA, Li H, et al. Comparison of the American-European Consensus Group Sjögren's syndrome classification criteria to newly proposed American College of Rheumatology criteria in a large, carefully characterised sicca cohort. Ann Rheum Dis 2014;73(1):31–8.
50. Cornec D, Jousse-Joulin S, Pers JO, et al. Contribution of salivary gland ultrasonography to the diagnosis of Sjögren's syndrome: toward new diagnostic criteria? Arthritis Rheum 2013;65(1):216–25.
51. Takagi Y, Sumi M, Nakamura H, et al. Ultrasonography as an additional item in the American College of Rheumatology classification of Sjögren's syndrome. Rheumatology (Oxford) 2014;53(11):1977–83.
52. Theander E, Mandl T. Primary Sjögren's syndrome: diagnostic and prognostic value of salivary gland ultrasonography using a simplified scoring system. Arthritis Care Res (Hoboken) 2014;66(7):1102–7.
53. Baldini C, Luciano N, Tarantini G, et al. Salivary gland ultrasonography: a highly specific tool for the early diagnosis of primary Sjögren's syndrome. Arthritis Res Ther 2015;17:146.
54. Luciano N, Baldini C, Tarantini G, et al. Ultrasonography of major salivary glands: a highly specific tool for distinguishing primary Sjögren's syndrome from undifferentiated connective tissue diseases. Rheumatology (Oxford) 2015;54(12): 2198–204.
55. Sun Z, Zhang Z, Fu K, et al. Diagnostic accuracy of parotid CT for identifying Sjögren's syndrome. Eur J Radiol 2012;81(10):2702–9.
56. Takashima S, Takeuchi N, Morimoto S, et al. MR imaging of Sjögren syndrome: correlation with sialography and pathology. J Comput Assist Tomogr 1991; 15(3):393–400.
57. Satoh M, Chan EK, Ho LA, et al. Prevalence and sociodemographic correlates of antinuclear antibodies in the United States. Arthritis Rheum 2012;64(7):2319–27.
58. Daniels TE, Cox D, Shiboski CH, et al. Associations between salivary gland histopathologic diagnoses and phenotypic features of Sjögren's syndrome among 1,726 registry participants. Arthritis Rheum 2011;63(7):2021–30.
59. Foulks GN, Forstot SL, Donshik PC, et al. Clinical guidelines for management of dry eye associated with Sjögren disease. Ocul Surf 2015;13(2):118–32.
60. Costantino D, Guaraldi C. Effectiveness and safety of vaginal suppositories for the treatment of the vaginal atrophy in postmenopausal women: an open, non-controlled clinical trial. Eur Rev Med Pharmacol Sci 2008;12(6):411–6.
61. Gottenberg JE, Ravaud P, Puechal X, et al. Effects of hydroxychloroquine on symptomatic improvement in primary Sjögren syndrome: the JOQUER randomized clinical trial. JAMA 2014;312(3):249–58.
62. Kruize AA, Hene RJ, Kallenberg CG, et al. Hydroxychloroquine treatment for primary Sjögren's syndrome: a two year double blind crossover trial. Ann Rheum Dis 1993;52(5):360–4.
63. Fox RI, Dixon R, Guarrasi V, et al. Treatment of primary Sjögren's syndrome with hydroxychloroquine: a retrospective, open-label study. Lupus 1996; 5(Suppl 1):S31–6.

64. Meijer JM, Meiners PM, Vissink A, et al. Effectiveness of rituximab treatment in primary Sjögren's syndrome: a randomized, double-blind, placebo-controlled trial. Arthritis Rheum 2010;62(4):960–8.

65. Devauchelle-Pensec V, Mariette X, Jousse-Joulin S, et al. Treatment of primary Sjögren syndrome with rituximab: a randomized trial. Ann Intern Med 2014; 160(4):233–42.

66. Carubbi F, Cipriani P, Marrelli A, et al. Efficacy and safety of rituximab treatment in early primary Sjögren's syndrome: a prospective, multi-center, follow-up study. Arthritis Res Ther 2013;15(5):R172.

Cardiovascular Disease Risk in Patients with Rheumatic Diseases

Rachel H. Mackey, PhD, MPH[a],*, Lewis H. Kuller, MD, DrPH[b],
Larry W. Moreland, MD[c]

KEYWORDS

- Rheumatoid arthritis • Cardiovascular • Lipids • Lipoproteins • Myocardial fibrosis

KEY POINTS

- Adults with rheumatoid arthritis (RA) have an ~1.5 times higher risk of cardiovascular disease (CVD) even with no traditional CVD risk factors, and incidence rates increase substantially with number of CVD risk factors.
- Low-density lipoprotein (LDL) or high-density lipoprotein (HDL) particles or apolipoproteins (apoB or apoA1) may be more reliable CVD risk factors than cholesterol (total, LDL-cholesterol, or HDL-cholesterol) concentrations because of chronic inflammation.
- In RA, current CVD risk factors likely underestimate the extent of subclinical atherosclerosis.
- Inflammation may directly cause myocardial injury and heart failure.
- Disease activity is a strong risk factor for CVD and mortality and key target for CVD risk reduction.

INTRODUCTION

Increased cardiovascular disease (CVD) risk has been reported for rheumatoid arthritis (RA) and other inflammatory autoimmune rheumatic diseases, which have a lifetime risk of adult onset of 1 in 12 for women and 1 in 20 for men.[1] This review focuses on the most common, RA, which occurs 2 to 3 times more often in women than men. The risk for CVD and total mortality is greater than 1.5 times higher in RA patients

---

Disclosure statement: Dr R.H. Mackey has received honoraria from the National Lipid Association related to educational, not promotional, endeavors. Dr L.W. Moreland serves on data safety monitoring boards for Boeringher-Ingelheim, Pfizer, and Acerta. None (Dr L.H. Kuller).
[a] Department of Epidemiology, University of Pittsburgh Graduate School of Public Health, University of Pittsburgh, 542 Bellefield Professional Building, 130 North Bellefield Avenue, Pittsburgh, PA 15213, USA; [b] Department of Epidemiology, University of Pittsburgh Graduate School of Public Health, Room 550, Bellefield Professional Building, 130 North Bellefield Avenue, Pittsburgh, PA 15213, USA; [c] Division of Rheumatology and Clinical Immunology, University of Pittsburgh School of Medicine, 3500 Terrace Street, Thomas E. Starzl Biomedical Science Tower South 711, Pittsburgh, PA 15261, USA
* Corresponding author.
E-mail address: mackey@edc.pitt.edu

and 10-year CVD risk scores underestimate risk. CVD is more likely to be fatal, and unrecognized myocardial infarctions (MI), sudden death, and heart failure (HF) are increased. More aggressive primary and secondary prevention of CVD is needed in RA patients,[2-4] many of whom are postmenopausal women. The current review focuses on the following (1) the role of dyslipidemia in RA-related CVD risk; (2) risk of inflammation-related myocardial disease and eventual HF; (3) the emergence of RA disease activity as a key focus for CVD risk prediction and CVD risk reduction in RA.

RA is associated with greater than 1.5-fold higher risk of coronary heart disease (CHD), CVD, HF,[5,6] venous thrombosis,[7,8] fatal CVD, and total mortality,[9-12] and other CVD outcomes (**Box 1**). Unrecognized MI, sudden death,[13] and asymptomatic HF[14,15] are all increased among RA patients.

The greater than 1.5-fold higher risk of CVD exists at most levels of traditional CVD risk factors, even among individuals with no smoking, diabetes, hypertension, or history of hypercholesterolemia, as shown in the Women's Health Initiative (WHI) RA Study (crude relative risk = 10.75/6.35 = 1.69) (**Table 1**).[16] CVD risk in RA is strongly related to traditional CVD risk factors, for example, cigarette smoking, hypertension, diabetes, and hyperlipidemia.[11,17-19] The risk factor profile in RA (**Box 2**) includes higher prevalence of smoking, hypertension,[20] diabetes,[17] and obesity, although some RA patients have low body mass index (BMI).

The role of dyslipidemia in RA has been questioned due to a "lipid paradox." RA patients have lower levels of total cholesterol (TC) and low-density lipoprotein (LDL) cholesterol (LDL-C) than adults without RA.[21] Increased CVD risk is associated with low levels of TC and LDL-C.[22] Total and LDL-C levels decrease before RA diagnosis,[23] often increase in response to anti-inflammatory medications, and decrease in response to flares of RA disease activity. The paradoxically low total and LDL-C levels contribute to underestimation of CVD risk by CVD risk scores (eg, Framingham Risk Score, Reynolds Risk Score,[24] and SCORE [Systematic COronary Risk Evaluation][25]), which have been shown to incorrectly classify as "low risk" approximately 60% of RA patients with coronary artery calcification greater than 300,[26] and approximately one-third of those who subsequently had CVD events.[25]

WHAT EXPLAINS THE EXCESS CARDIOVASCULAR DISEASE RISK IN RHEUMATOID ARTHRITIS?

Active RA is characterized by systemic inflammation that is credited with much of the excess risk of CVD and mortality in RA. The contribution of inflammation to

---

Box 1
Cardiovascular diseases increased in rheumatoid arthritis

- Myocardial infarction (often unrecognized)[13]
- Sudden death[13]
- Stroke[9]
- Venous thrombosis[7,8]
- Heart failure[5,6]
- Diastolic dysfunction[65]
- Peripheral vascular disease[78]
- Subclinical atherosclerosis[72,79,80]
- Endothelial dysfunction[81]

Table 1
Weighted age-adjusted cardiovascular disease incidence rate (per 1000 person-years) among the Women's Health Initiative participants by risk factor combinations and groups of women with rheumatoid arthritis, with unverified rheumatoid arthritis, or not reporting rheumatoid arthritis[a]

	All Women with RA (Anti-CCP-Positive and/or Taking DMARDs)	Women with Unverified RA (Anti-CCP-Negative and Not Taking DMARDs)	Women with No Reported RA
No smoking, hypertension, diabetes mellitus, or high cholesterol			
Incidence (95% CI)	10.75 (5.75–20.89)[b,c]	8.28 (6.14–11.20)	6.35 (5.94–6.78)
No./total no. of events	25/217	125/1320	2480/36,299
Smoking only			
Incidence (95% CI)	16.99 (10.83–26.78)[b,c]	10.50 (8.09–13.65)	8.18 (7.72–8.66)
No./total no. of events	56/327	163/1445	3446/41,205
Hypertension only			
Incidence (95% CI)	16.99 (8.13–37.74)	15.36 (11.77–20.20)	12.53 (11.72–13.41)
No./total no. of events	19/106	161/907	2540/17,297
Hypertension and smoking only			
Incidence (95% CI)	27.35 (16.80–45.21)[b,c]	18.50 (14.39–23.84)	16.59 (15.63–17.61)
No./total no. of events	45/179	186/941	3253/18,041
Diabetes mellitus and hypertension only			
Incidence (95% CI)	45.72 (10.98–216.51)	37.77 (22.09–65.29)	27.03 (23.14–31.60)
No./total no. of events	5/16	43/124	477/1746

[a] Excluding those with CVD at baseline or RA only at follow-up.
[b] $P<.05$ versus women with unverified RA.
[c] $P<.05$ versus women with no reported RA.
From Mackey RH, Kuller LH, Deane KD, et al. Rheumatoid arthritis, anti-cyclic citrullinated peptide positivity, and cardiovascular disease risk in the Women's Health Initiative. Arthritis Rheumatol 2015;67(9):2315; with permission.

atherosclerosis, endothelial dysfunction, plaque vulnerability, and atherothrombotic events has been previously reviewed.[27,28] Reduction of CVD risk has been reported using several anti-inflammatory disease-modifying antirheumatic drugs (DMARDs), including hydroxychloroquine[29] and methotrexate,[30] and possibly for biological medications such as tumor necrosis factor (TNF-α) inhibitors.[31] Randomized clinical trials are underway, testing methotrexate[27] and an anti-interleukin (IL)-1β antibody (canakinumab) for secondary prevention of CVD events among adults without RA.[27] RA-associated inflammation also contributes to the development of dysfunctional high-density lipoprotein (HDL) as recently reviewed.[32] Primary and secondary prevention of CVD may be suboptimal in RA patients, most of whom are postmenopausal women without elevated LDL-C.[2–4]

The current review focuses on the following issues: (1) reconsideration of the role of dyslipidemia in CVD risk; (2) potential role of inflammation on myocardial disease and eventual HF; and (3) emerging role of disease activity as key for CVD risk prediction and CVD risk reduction in RA.

> **Box 2**
> **Cardiovascular disease risk factors in rheumatoid arthritis patients**
>
> *Traditional*
>
> - ↑ Smoking, past, current
> - ↑ Hypertension
> - ↑ Diabetes
> - ↓ Total and LDL-cholesterol (sometimes with ↓ HDL-cholesterol and ↑ triglycerides)
> - ↓ Physical activity
> - ↑ Obesity and ↓ low BMI
> - ↑ Inflammation (CRP, ESR, cytokines)
>
> *Possible*
>
> - ↑ Dysfunctional HDL
> - ↑ ApoB, LDL-P
> - ↑ Lipoprotein(a)

ROLE OF DYSLIPIDEMIA IN CARDIOVASCULAR DISEASE RISK IN RHEUMATOID ARTHRITIS

Can Lipoprotein Particle Concentrations Explain the Lipid Paradox in Rheumatoid Arthritis?

The "lipid paradox" in RA describes the seemingly paradoxic association of low levels of total and LDL cholesterol with increased CVD risk.[22] However, recent large studies show a J-shaped association of LDL-C with CVD in RA,[33,34] that is similar to non-RA controls.[34] Indeed, the lipid paradox of high CVD risk with normal or low LDL-C is well known in adults with the metabolic syndrome, diabetes, or obesity. These conditions are characterized by increased levels of inflammation, triglycerides, and small, dense, cholesterol-depleted LDL particles (LDL-P) that result in increased levels of LDL-P levels despite decreased levels of LDL-cholesterol (LDL-C) levels. LDL-P can be measured directly or estimated by ApoB concentration, because there is one apoB per LDL and very LDL particle, and ∼90% are LDL-P. When discordance exists between concentrations of atherogenic lipoproteins (eg, apoB, LDL-P) and their cholesterol content (LDL-C or non-HDL-C), CVD risk is better estimated using particle concentrations rather than cholesterol level, as demonstrated in the Multi-Ethnic Study of Atherosclerosis (**Fig. 1**) and other studies.[35–38] The effect of HDL on CVD risk is much more complicated. Increasing evidence suggests that CVD risk and HDL functionality are more related to concentrations of HDL particles (HDL-P) and apoA1 than HDL cholesterol.[39]

Measurements of apoB, LDL-P, apoA1, and HDL-P may be useful in CVD risk assessment. In many studies, apoB or the apoB/apoA1 ratio is independently associated with CVD risk when total and LDL-C are not[40,41] and are also associated with progression of atherosclerosis in the carotid[42] and coronary arteries.[43] Recent studies also suggest that LDL-P > LDL-C or apoB > LDL-C discordance is common in RA. Several studies report that compared with controls, RA patients have higher levels of small LDL-P,[44,45] and higher levels of apoB (and triglycerides) despite similar LDL-C levels,[43,46] similar levels of LDL-P, or lower levels of LDL-C[47] (ie, apoB > LDL-C or LDLP > LDL-C discordance). Measuring lipoprotein particles or

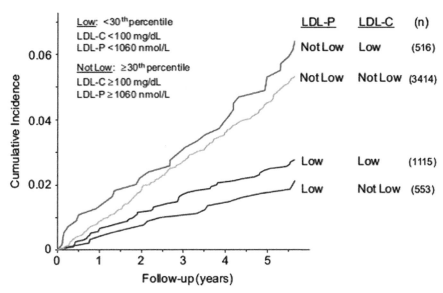

Fig. 1. Cumulative incidence of cardiovascular events in subgroups with low LDL-C and/or low LDL-P, from proportional hazards models adjusted for age and gender. Low LDL-C and LDL-P values were defined as less than 100 mg/dL and less than 1060 nmol/L, respectively (<30th percentile). (*From* Otvos JD, Mora S, Shalaurova I, et al. Clinical implications of discordance between low-density lipoprotein cholesterol and particle number. J Clin Lipidol 2011;5(2):110; with permission.)

apolipoproteins will provide more reliable information regarding risk and effects of disease activity and medications. Equivalent population cut points for LDL-C, non-HDL-C, LDL-P, and apoB have been described.[48] More importantly, these results emphasize the role of dyslipidemia in RA. For this reason, statin therapy, which reduces LDL-P, apoB, and LDL-C levels[49] and reduces CVD events in adults with low LDL-C but elevated C-reactive protein (CRP),[50] is very important adjunct therapy in RA patients. Recent recommendations for dyslipidemia management from the National Lipid Association specifically address RA.[51,52] Recommendations include counting RA is as an additional atherosclerotic cardiovascular disease risk factor for risk stratification, rechecking LDL-C levels after RA flare, and using non-HDL-C, apoB, or LDL particle concentration instead of LDL-C when discordance exists.[51]

Current Risk Factors in Rheumatoid Arthritis Patients Underestimate Prior Exposures and Burden of Atherosclerosis

Among RA patients, current levels of smoking, lipids, BMI, and other risk factors underestimate CVD risk. A substantial portion of this unexplained excess risk appears related to an accelerated burden of subclinical atherosclerosis that develops before the clinical features of RA. CVD risk is substantially increased by the time RA is diagnosed[19] and even before diagnosis, with a 3-fold higher chance of MI in the 2 years before diagnosis.[13] One study showed that dyslipidemia may be increased pre-RA. Ten years before the diagnosis of RA, individuals who develop RA have higher levels of apoB (6%, +0.06 g/L), TC (4%, +8.1 mg/dL), triglycerides (17%, +46.9 mg/dL), and lower HDL-C (−9%) than individuals who did not develop RA.[53] Another study showed that in the 5 years before RA diagnosis, levels of total and LDL-C decreased, but levels of triglycerides, a strong predictor of higher apoB and LDL-P levels, did not.[23]

Substantially Increased Burden of Atherosclerosis at Diagnosis of Rheumatoid Arthritis?

Increased subclinical atherosclerosis compared with controls is seen in early RA,[54,55] with faster progression of carotid intima-media thickness (cIMT) in early RA versus late RA[56] and a similar prevalence of carotid plaques for early versus late RA. One study showed that the extent of calcified plaque in the aorta and coronary and carotid arteries is more than 10 years ahead of non-RA controls (**Fig. 2**).[57] Among RA patients, even among those aged less than 40 years, 50% of RA patients had calcified plaque in a least 1 of the 3 vascular sites. The presence of calcified plaque increased to 75% for those ages 50 to 60 and greater than 90% for those aged greater than 60 years. These results are especially striking given that other studies show that, in RA, noncalcified plaque (not detected by these measures and thought to be more vulnerable) is more common than calcified plaque.[58]

Inflammation May Cause Myocardial Disease Directly, Leading to Heart Failure

The risk of HF in RA is increased more than 2-fold and is poorly explained by CVD risk factors or ischemic heart disease.[59] One study showed increased myocardial ischemia levels in RA patients without evidence of obstructive coronary artery disease.[60] Inflammatory markers that are increased in RA (eg, erythrocyte sedimentation rate [ESR], CRP, white blood cell count, and cytokines, including IL-6 and TNF-α) have stronger associations with fatal CVD, mortality, and HF than with atherosclerosis and MI.[61–63] Evidence suggests that inflammation contributes to myocardial microvascular endothelial dysfunction, remodeling, interstitial fibrosis, and diastolic dysfunction, leading to HF, specifically with preserved ejection fraction (HFPEF).[64] HF in RA is more often HFPEF, and fatal,[15] and RA is associated with diastolic dysfunction,[65]

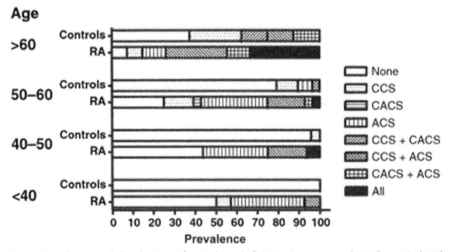

Fig. 2. Prevalence and distribution of vascular calcification in coronary (CACS), aortic (ACS), and carotid arteries (CCS) by age in control subjects and patients with rheumatoid arthritis. (*From* Wang S, Yiu KH, Mok MY, et al. Prevalence and extent of calcification over aorta, coronary and carotid arteries in patients with rheumatoid arthritis. J Intern Med 2009;266(5):449; with permission.)

left ventricular concentric remodeling,[66] and reduced left ventricular mass.[67] Levels of myocardial fibrosis and inflammation are increased in RA patients when measured with cardiac MRI[68,69] and are associated with myocardial dysfunction and higher RA disease activity.[68,69] Future assessments of anti-inflammatory medications and other RA interventions will likely include measures of subclinical myocardial fibrosis and damage.

Emergence of Rheumatoid Arthritis Disease Activity as Key Predictor and Target for Prevention of Cardiovascular Disease Risk

RA treatment seeks to reduce disease activity, assessed using various scores based on numbers of swollen and tender joints, with or without inflammatory markers such as ESR or CRP. Increasing evidence indicates that reducing RA disease activity is critical for CVD risk prevention. Several recent RA studies showed strong associations of cumulative exposure to disease activity, "flares" of disease activity, and joint pain, with increased CVD risk.[70,71] Most importantly, with anti-IL-6 treatment, greater reductions in disease activity and swollen and tender joint counts were independently related to lower CVD risk during follow-up.[71] Inflammation may explain the association of higher disease activity with higher cIMT,[72] development of new carotid plaque, progression of carotid plaque over 3 years,[56] and with coronary[58] and carotid plaque vulnerability.[73] Disease activity may also increase CVD risk via effects of joint symptoms on physical activity and ability to adhere to certain types of risk factor modification.[74] Interrelationships of disease activity, inflammation and joint pain may explain results from the WHI-RA Study showing that joint pain severity was associated with higher CHD incidence among postmenopausal women with RA, but also among women with unspecified arthritis, and among the general population of women without RA or arthritis.[16]

A new RA-specific CVD risk calculator (ERS-RA [Extended Risk Score- Rheumatoid Arthritis]) found, in addition to traditional CVD risk factors, the following added to risk prediction: disease activity (clinical disease activity index, which does not include CRP or other inflammation markers), disability (Health Assessment Questionnaire), disease duration greater than 10 years, and prednisone use.[75] In contrast, seropositivity (antibodies to cyclic citrullinated peptides (anti-CCP or ACPA)+ or Rheumatoid Factor [RF] +), erosions, and subcutaneous nodules were not significantly associated with CVD risk. Since RA-specific CVD risk factors (**Box 3**) are also associated with increased RA disease severity, these results suggest that RA disease activity and severity may substantially account for their associations with CVD risk. However, anti-CCP+ and RF+ may be directly related to HF and total mortality through effects on lungs or

---

Box 3
Rheumatoid arthritis–specific cardiovascular disease risk factors

- Disease activity (scores of joint pain, inflammation)
- Disease duration (>10 years)
- Seropositivity (anti-CCP+ or RF+)
- Rheumatoid nodules
- Extra-articular disease
- Inflammatory markers
- HLA shared epitope

kidneys. For example, over a 36-year follow-up in the Nurses' Health Study, respiratory mortality was increased among women with seropositive RA (hazard ratio 2.67, 95% confidence interval [CI] 1.89–3.77), but not for seronegative RA, compared with women without RA.[76] Although that study did not have information on DMARD exposure or disease activity, the results agree with a report of greater immune cell accumulation and activation in lung tissue of anti-CCP + RA versus anti-CCP-RA and controls.[77]

SUMMARY

The risk of CVD and death is substantially increased among adults with RA, most of whom are postmenopausal women. Current risk factor levels, especially total and LDL-C and smoking, and CVD risk scores underestimate their risk due to an accelerated burden of subclinical atherosclerosis. Aggressive management and control of risk factors, that is, smoking cessation, antihypertensive and lipid-lowering medications, is needed, at earlier ages. Reducing disease activity and inflammation may be essential for reducing myocardial disease and fibrosis of the heart, lung, and kidney. Further evaluation with new imaging techniques are needed to determine effects of anti-inflammatory drugs on myocardial, lung, and kidney fibrosis. Ongoing clinical trials of anti-inflammatory medications will provide important evidence about whether reducing inflammation will reduce the risk of CHD, CVD, and total mortality.

REFERENCES

1. Crowson CS, Matteson EL, Myasoedova E, et al. The lifetime risk of adult-onset rheumatoid arthritis and other inflammatory autoimmune rheumatic diseases. Arthritis Rheum 2011;63:633–9.
2. Toms TE, Panoulas VF, Douglas KM, et al. Statin use in rheumatoid arthritis in relation to actual cardiovascular risk: evidence for substantial undertreatment of lipid-associated cardiovascular risk? Ann Rheum Dis 2010;69:683–8.
3. Bartels CM, Kind AJ, Thorpe CT, et al. Lipid testing in patients with rheumatoid arthritis and key cardiovascular-related comorbidities: a medicare analysis. Semin Arthritis Rheum 2012;42:9–16.
4. Bartels CM, Saucier JM, Thorpe CT, et al. Monitoring diabetes in patients with and without rheumatoid arthritis: a medicare study. Arthritis Res Ther 2012;14:R166.
5. Nicola PJ, Maradit-Kremers H, Roger VL, et al. The risk of congestive heart failure in rheumatoid arthritis: a population-based study over 46 years. Arthritis Rheum 2005;52:412–20.
6. Nicola PJ, Crowson CS, Maradit-Kremers H, et al. Contribution of congestive heart failure and ischemic heart disease to excess mortality in rheumatoid arthritis. Arthritis Rheum 2006;54:60–7.
7. Bacani AK, Gabriel SE, Crowson CS, et al. Noncardiac vascular disease in rheumatoid arthritis: increase in venous thromboembolic events? Arthritis Rheum 2012;64:53–61.
8. Holmqvist ME, Neovius M, Eriksson J, et al. Risk of venous thromboembolism in patients with rheumatoid arthritis and association with disease duration and hospitalization. JAMA 2012;308:1350–6.
9. Meune C, Touze E, Trinquart L, et al. High risk of clinical cardiovascular events in rheumatoid arthritis: levels of associations of myocardial infarction and stroke through a systematic review and meta-analysis. Arch Cardiovasc Dis 2010;103: 253–61.

10. Avina-Zubieta JA, Choi HK, Sadatsafavi M, et al. Risk of cardiovascular mortality in patients with rheumatoid arthritis: a meta-analysis of observational studies. Arthritis Rheum 2008;59:1690–7.

11. Solomon DH, Karlson EW, Rimm EB, et al. Cardiovascular morbidity and mortality in women diagnosed with rheumatoid arthritis. Circulation 2003;107:1303–7.

12. Meune C, Touze E, Trinquart L, et al. Trends in cardiovascular mortality in patients with rheumatoid arthritis over 50 years: a systematic review and meta-analysis of cohort studies. Rheumatology (Oxford) 2009;48:1309–13.

13. Maradit-Kremers H, Crowson CS, Nicola PJ, et al. Increased unrecognized coronary heart disease and sudden deaths in rheumatoid arthritis: a population-based cohort study. Arthritis Rheum 2005;52:402–11.

14. Bhatia GS, Sosin MD, Patel JV, et al. Left ventricular systolic dysfunction in rheumatoid disease: an unrecognized burden? J Am Coll Cardiol 2006;47:1169–74.

15. Davis JM 3rd, Roger VL, Crowson CS, et al. The presentation and outcome of heart failure in patients with rheumatoid arthritis differs from that in the general population. Arthritis Rheum 2008;58:2603–11.

16. Mackey RH, Kuller LH, Deane KD, et al. Rheumatoid arthritis, anti-cyclic citrullinated peptide positivity, and cardiovascular disease risk in the women's health initiative. Arthritis Rheumatol 2015;67:2311–22.

17. Boyer JF, Gourraud PA, Cantagrel A, et al. Traditional cardiovascular risk factors in rheumatoid arthritis: a meta-analysis. Joint Bone Spine 2011;78:179–83.

18. Solomon DH, Curhan GC, Rimm EB, et al. Cardiovascular risk factors in women with and without rheumatoid arthritis. Arthritis Rheum 2004;50:3444–9.

19. Kremers HM, Crowson CS, Therneau TM, et al. High ten-year risk of cardiovascular disease in newly diagnosed rheumatoid arthritis patients: a population-based cohort study. Arthritis Rheum 2008;58:2268–74.

20. Chung CP, Giles JT, Petri M, et al. Prevalence of traditional modifiable cardiovascular risk factors in patients with rheumatoid arthritis: comparison with control subjects from the multi-ethnic study of atherosclerosis. Semin Arthritis Rheum 2012;41:535–44.

21. Liao KP, Cai T, Gainer VS, et al. Lipid and lipoprotein levels and trend in rheumatoid arthritis compared to the general population. Arthritis Care Res (Hoboken) 2013;65:2046–50.

22. Myasoedova E, Crowson CS, Kremers HM, et al. Lipid paradox in rheumatoid arthritis: the impact of serum lipid measures and systemic inflammation on the risk of cardiovascular disease. Ann Rheum Dis 2011;70:482–7.

23. Myasoedova E, Crowson CS, Kremers HM, et al. Total cholesterol and LDL levels decrease before rheumatoid arthritis. Ann Rheum Dis 2010;69:1310–4.

24. Crowson CS, Matteson EL, Roger VL, et al. Usefulness of risk scores to estimate the risk of cardiovascular disease in patients with rheumatoid arthritis. Am J Cardiol 2012;110:420–4.

25. Arts EE, Popa C, Den Broeder AA, et al. Performance of four current risk algorithms in predicting cardiovascular events in patients with early rheumatoid arthritis. Ann Rheum Dis 2015;74(4):668–74.

26. Kawai VK, Chung CP, Solus JF, et al. The ability of the 2013 American College of Cardiology/American Heart Association cardiovascular risk score to identify rheumatoid arthritis patients with high coronary artery calcification scores. Arthritis Rheumatol 2015;67:381–5.

27. Ridker PM. Testing the inflammatory hypothesis of atherothrombosis: scientific rationale for the cardiovascular inflammation reduction trial (CIRT). J Thromb Haemost 2009;7(Suppl 1):332–9.

28. Ridker PM. From C-reactive protein to interleukin-6 to interleukin-1: moving upstream to identify novel targets for atheroprotection. Circ Res 2016;118:145–56.

29. Sharma TS, Wasko MC, Tang X, et al. Hydroxychloroquine use is associated with decreased incident cardiovascular events in rheumatoid arthritis patients. J Am Heart Assoc 2016;5:e002867.

30. Micha R, Imamura F, Wyler von Ballmoos M, et al. Systematic review and meta-analysis of methotrexate use and risk of cardiovascular disease. Am J Cardiol 2011;108:1362–70.

31. Barnabe C, Martin BJ, Ghali WA. Systematic review and meta-analysis: anti-tumor necrosis factor alpha therapy and cardiovascular events in rheumatoid arthritis. Arthritis Care Res (Hoboken) 2011;63:522–9.

32. Ormseth MJ, Stein CM. High-density lipoprotein function in rheumatoid arthritis. Curr Opin Lipidol 2016;27:67–75.

33. Zhang J, Chen L, Delzell E, et al. The association between inflammatory markers, serum lipids and the risk of cardiovascular events in patients with rheumatoid arthritis. Ann Rheum Dis 2014;73:1301–8.

34. Liao KP, Liu J, Lu B, et al. Association between lipid levels and major adverse cardiovascular events in rheumatoid arthritis compared to non-rheumatoid arthritis patients. Arthritis Rheumatol 2015;67:2004–10.

35. Otvos JD, Mora S, Shalaurova I, et al. Clinical implications of discordance between low-density lipoprotein cholesterol and particle number. J Clin Lipidol 2011;5:105–13.

36. Sniderman AD, Islam S, Yusuf S, et al. Discordance analysis of apolipoprotein b and non-high density lipoprotein cholesterol as markers of cardiovascular risk in the Interheart Study. Atherosclerosis 2012;225:444–9.

37. Pencina MJ, D'Agostino RB, Zdrojewski T, et al. Apolipoprotein b improves risk assessment of future coronary heart disease in the Framingham Heart Study beyond LDL-c and non-HDL-c. Eur J Prev Cardiol 2015;22:1321–7.

38. Wilkins JT, Li RC, Sniderman A, et al. Discordance between apolipoprotein b and LDL-cholesterol in young adults predicts coronary artery calcification: the Cardia study. J Am Coll Cardiol 2016;67:193–201.

39. Mackey RH, Greenland P, Goff DC Jr, et al. High-density lipoprotein cholesterol and particle concentrations, carotid atherosclerosis, and coronary events: MESA (Multi-Ethnic Study of Atherosclerosis). J Am Coll Cardiol 2012;60:508–16.

40. Rao VU, Pavlov A, Klearman M, et al. An evaluation of risk factors for major adverse cardiovascular events during tocilizumab therapy. Arthritis Rheumatol 2015;67:372–80.

41. Ohman M, Ohman ML, Wallberg-Jonsson S. The apoB/apoA1 ratio predicts future cardiovascular events in patients with rheumatoid arthritis. Scand J Rheumatol 2014;43:259–64.

42. Ajeganova S, Ehrnfelt C, Alizadeh R, et al. Longitudinal levels of apolipoproteins and antibodies against phosphorylcholine are independently associated with carotid artery atherosclerosis 5 years after rheumatoid arthritis onset–a prospective cohort study. Rheumatology (Oxford) 2011;50:1785–93.

43. Knowlton N, Wages JA, Centola MB, et al. Apolipoprotein b-containing lipoprotein subclasses as risk factors for cardiovascular disease in patients with rheumatoid arthritis. Arthritis Care Res (Hoboken) 2012;64:993–1000.

44. Hurt-Camejo E, Paredes S, Masana L, et al. Elevated levels of small, low-density lipoprotein with high affinity for arterial matrix components in patients with rheumatoid arthritis: possible contribution of phospholipase a2 to this atherogenic profile. Arthritis Rheum 2001;44:2761–7.

45. Rizzo M, Spinas GA, Cesur M, et al. Atherogenic lipoprotein phenotype and LDL size and subclasses in drug-naive patients with early rheumatoid arthritis. Atherosclerosis 2009;207:502–6.
46. Choi HK, Seeger JD. Lipid profiles among us elderly with untreated rheumatoid arthritis–the third national health and nutrition examination survey. J Rheumatol 2005;32:2311–6.
47. Charles-Schoeman C, Fleischmann R, Davignon J, et al. Potential mechanisms leading to the abnormal lipid profile in patients with rheumatoid arthritis versus healthy volunteers and reversal by tofacitinib. Arthritis Rheumatol 2015;67: 616–25.
48. Contois JH, McConnell JP, Sethi AA, et al. Apolipoprotein b and cardiovascular disease risk: position statement from the AACC lipoproteins and vascular diseases division working group on best practices. Clin Chem 2009;55:407–19.
49. Rosenson RS, Otvos JD, Hsia J. Effects of rosuvastatin and atorvastatin on LDL and HDL particle concentrations in patients with metabolic syndrome: a randomized, double-blind, controlled study. Diabetes Care 2009;32:1087–91.
50. Ridker PM, Danielson E, Fonseca FA, et al. Rosuvastatin to prevent vascular events in men and women with elevated c-reactive protein. N Engl J Med 2008;359:2195–207.
51. Jacobson TA, Maki KC, Orringer CE, et al. National Lipid Association recommendations for patient-centered management of dyslipidemia: part 2. J Clin Lipidol 2015;9:S1–122.e1.
52. Jacobson TA, Ito MK, Maki KC, et al. National Lipid Association recommendations for patient-centered management of dyslipidemia: part 1—executive summary. J Clin Lipidol 2014;8:473–88.
53. van Halm VP, Nielen MM, Nurmohamed MT, et al. Lipids and inflammation: serial measurements of the lipid profile of blood donors who later developed rheumatoid arthritis. Ann Rheum Dis 2007;66:184–8.
54. Hannawi S, Haluska B, Marwick TH, et al. Atherosclerotic disease is increased in recent-onset rheumatoid arthritis: a critical role for inflammation. Arthritis Res Ther 2007;9:R116.
55. Ambrosino P, Lupoli R, Di Minno A, et al. Subclinical atherosclerosis in patients with rheumatoid arthritis. A meta-analysis of literature studies. Thromb Haemost 2015;113:916–30.
56. Giles JT, Post WS, Blumenthal RS, et al. Longitudinal predictors of progression of carotid atherosclerosis in rheumatoid arthritis. Arthritis Rheum 2011;63:3216–25.
57. Wang S, Yiu KH, Mok MY, et al. Prevalence and extent of calcification over aorta, coronary and carotid arteries in patients with rheumatoid arthritis. J Intern Med 2009;266:445–52.
58. Karpouzas GA, Malpeso J, Choi TY, et al. Prevalence, extent and composition of coronary plaque in patients with rheumatoid arthritis without symptoms or prior diagnosis of coronary artery disease. Ann Rheum Dis 2014;73(10):1797–804.
59. Crowson CS, Nicola PJ, Kremers HM, et al. How much of the increased incidence of heart failure in rheumatoid arthritis is attributable to traditional cardiovascular risk factors and ischemic heart disease? Arthritis Rheum 2005;52:3039–44.
60. Toutouzas K, Sfikakis PP, Karanasos A, et al. Myocardial ischaemia without obstructive coronary artery disease in rheumatoid arthritis: hypothesis-generating insights from a cross-sectional study. Rheumatology (Oxford) 2013; 52:76–80.
61. Ajeganova S, Andersson ML, Frostegard J, et al. Disease factors in early rheumatoid arthritis are associated with differential risks for cardiovascular events and

mortality depending on age at onset: a 10-year observational cohort study. J Rheumatol 2013;40:1958–66.

62. Maradit-Kremers H, Nicola PJ, Crowson CS, et al. Cardiovascular death in rheumatoid arthritis: a population-based study. Arthritis Rheum 2005;52:722–32.

63. Maradit-Kremers H, Nicola PJ, Crowson CS, et al. Raised erythrocyte sedimentation rate signals heart failure in patients with rheumatoid arthritis. Ann Rheum Dis 2007;66:76–80.

64. Paulus WJ, Tschope C. A novel paradigm for heart failure with preserved ejection fraction: comorbidities drive myocardial dysfunction and remodeling through coronary microvascular endothelial inflammation. J Am Coll Cardiol 2013;62:263–71.

65. Aslam F, Bandeali SJ, Khan NA, et al. Diastolic dysfunction in rheumatoid arthritis: a meta-analysis and systematic review. Arthritis Care Res (Hoboken) 2013;65: 534–43.

66. Myasoedova E, Davis JM 3rd, Crowson CS, et al. Brief report: rheumatoid arthritis is associated with left ventricular concentric remodeling: results of a population-based cross-sectional study. Arthritis Rheum 2013;65:1713–8.

67. Giles JT, Malayeri AA, Fernandes V, et al. Left ventricular structure and function in patients with rheumatoid arthritis, as assessed by cardiac magnetic resonance imaging. Arthritis Rheum 2010;62:940–51.

68. Kobayashi Y, Giles JT, Hirano M, et al. Assessment of myocardial abnormalities in rheumatoid arthritis using a comprehensive cardiac magnetic resonance approach: a pilot study. Arthritis Res Ther 2010;12:R171.

69. Ntusi NA, Piechnik SK, Francis JM, et al. Diffuse myocardial fibrosis and inflammation in rheumatoid arthritis: insights from CMR t1 mapping. JACC Cardiovasc Imaging 2015;8:526–36.

70. Myasoedova E, Chandran A, Ilhan B, et al. The role of rheumatoid arthritis (RA) flare and cumulative burden of ra severity in the risk of cardiovascular disease. Ann Rheum Dis 2016;75(3):560–5.

71. Rider OJ, Lewis AJ, Lewandowski AJ, et al. Obese subjects show sex-specific differences in right ventricular hypertrophy. Circ Cardiovasc Imaging 2014;8(1).

72. van Sijl AM, Peters MJ, Knol DK, et al. Carotid intima media thickness in rheumatoid arthritis as compared to control subjects: a meta-analysis. Semin Arthritis Rheum 2011;40:389–97.

73. Semb AG, Rollefstad S, Provan SA, et al. Carotid plaque characteristics and disease activity in rheumatoid arthritis. J Rheumatol 2013;40:359–68.

74. Akkara Veetil BM, Myasoedova E, Matteson EL, et al. Use of lipid-lowering agents in rheumatoid arthritis: a population-based cohort study. J Rheumatol 2013;40: 1082–8.

75. Solomon DH, Greenberg J, Curtis JR, et al. Derivation and internal validation of an expanded cardiovascular risk prediction score for rheumatoid arthritis: a consortium of rheumatology researchers of North America Registry Study. Arthritis Rheumatol 2015;67:1995–2003.

76. Sparks JA, Chang SC, Liao KP, et al. Rheumatoid arthritis and mortality among women during 36 years of prospective follow-up: results from the Nurses' Health Study. Arthritis Care Res (Hoboken) 2016;68(6):753–62.

77. Reynisdottir G, Karimi R, Joshua V, et al. Structural changes and antibody enrichment in the lungs are early features of anti-citrullinated protein antibody-positive rheumatoid arthritis. Arthritis Rheumatol 2014;66:31–9.

78. Stamatelopoulos KS, Kitas GD, Papamichael CM, et al. Subclinical peripheral arterial disease in rheumatoid arthritis. Atherosclerosis 2010;212:305–9.

79. Tyrrell PN, Beyene J, Feldman BM, et al. Rheumatic disease and carotid intima-media thickness: a systematic review and meta-analysis. Arterioscler Thromb Vasc Biol 2010;30:1014–26.
80. Kao AH, Krishnaswami S, Cunningham A, et al. Subclinical coronary artery calcification and relationship to disease duration in women with rheumatoid arthritis. J Rheumatol 2008;35:61–9.
81. Di Minno MN, Ambrosino P, Lupoli R, et al. Clinical assessment of endothelial function in patients with rheumatoid arthritis: a meta-analysis of literature studies. Eur J Intern Med 2015;26:835–42.

Gaps in Aging Research as it Applies to Rheumatologic Clinical Care

Una E. Makris, MD, MSc[a],*, Devyani Misra, MD, MSc[b],
Raymond Yung, MD, MB, ChB[c]

KEYWORDS

- Older adults • Rheumatology • Barriers • Education • Research

KEY POINTS

- The incidence and prevalence of rheumatologic diseases (including osteoarthritis, rheumatoid arthritis, systemic lupus erythematosus, and polymyalgia rheumatica) are increasing and the rheumatology workforce must be aware of aging-specific issues.
- Understanding the biology of aging and aging-related mechanisms that underlie rheumatologic diseases may help identify treatment targets and improve outcomes for older adults.
- Older adults pose unique challenges to the assessment and management of rheumatologic disease because this population often has multimorbidity, polypharmacy, frailty, cognitive impairment, and fragmented social support systems.
- An effective approach to older adults with rheumatologic conditions requires a better understanding of the mechanisms underlying the disease, time horizons and expectations of the patient, and outcomes that are mutually relevant to patient and provider.
- Training rheumatologists in principles of geriatric medicine, and geriatricians in musculoskeletal health as it applies to an aging population, will be critical.

By 2030, the size of the 65 years and older age group is expected to reach 71.5 million, or 20% of the total US population. Most of the older population is projected to be between age 65 and 74 years until 2034, when all of the baby boomers will be more than 70 years old.[1] By extension, the number of older adults with degenerative and

Disclosure: The authors have nothing to disclose.
[a] Division of Rheumatic Diseases, Department of Internal Medicine, UT Southwestern Medical Center and the VA North Texas Health Care System, 5323 Harry Hines Boulevard, Dallas, TX 75390-9169, USA; [b] Section of Clinical Epidemiology, Department of Medicine, Boston University School of Medicine, 650 Albany Street, Suite X-200, Boston, MA 02118, USA; [c] Division of Geriatric and Palliative Medicine, Department of Internal Medicine, VA Ann Arbor Health System, University of Michigan, 914 NIB, North Ingalls, Ann Arbor, MI 48109-0940, USA
* Corresponding author.
E-mail address: una.makris@utsouthwestern.edu

Clin Geriatr Med 33 (2017) 119–133
http://dx.doi.org/10.1016/j.cger.2016.08.009
0749-0690/17/Published by Elsevier Inc.

inflammatory rheumatologic diseases will increase in the subsequent decades and both the rheumatology and geriatric medicine workforce must be prepared to manage these conditions.

Osteoarthritis (OA), a degenerative joint disease commonly affecting hands, knees, hip, and spine, is the most common source of chronic joint pain among older adults. Estimates from 2005 suggest that OA affects approximately 27 million people in the United States alone.[2] Because age is a major risk factor for OA, its incidence and prevalence is expected to increase with aging of the population.[3] Besides OA, advanced age is also associated with a higher incidence and prevalence of inflammatory rheumatologic diseases, such as rheumatoid arthritis (RA), systemic lupus erythematosus (SLE), polymyalgia rheumatica (PMR), and giant cell arteritis (GCA). The incidence of RA continues to increase until age 75 to 80 years.[4] Although SLE is an autoimmune multisystem disease that most commonly affects women of child-bearing age, up to 18% of cases have an onset after age 50 years.[5] There are conflicting data regarding whether late-onset SLE has a more benign clinical course than SLE in younger populations.[6,7] Some reports suggest lower disease severity in late-onset SLE compared with younger patients with SLE.[6] Other research suggests greater disease activity and damage, and poorer survival; these findings are likely caused by greater frequency of comorbid conditions and greater organ damage at the time of diagnosis.[5] Rheumatologic diseases such as PMR and GCA exclusively affect older adults. Although the exact mechanisms leading to the development of PMR and GCA remain unclear, aging-related changes in the innate and adaptive immune systems are implicated.[8]

The reasons underlying the increasing incidence of these rheumatologic diseases in older age, especially for those conditions traditionally thought to affect mostly younger populations, are not fully understood. Rheumatologists' primary goals are to maintain function, reduce progression to chronic deformities, and minimize toxicity from therapy. Furthermore, these diseases may manifest very differently in older populations than in younger populations. In addition, clinicians still have much to learn about the process of aging and its impact on rheumatologic diseases. In 2014, a seminal publication by the Trans- National Institutes of Health (NIH) Geroscience Interest Group outlined what they called 7 pillars of aging discussed how these biological processes intersect and connect with chronic disease.[9] Although not specifically focused on rheumatologic disease, many of these pillars and the mechanistic relationships between aging and chronic diseases can be applied to clinical rheumatology. For example, the pillars of inflammation, epigenetics, adaptation to stress, and proteostasis are all known or suspected to play prominent roles, to different degrees, in rheumatologic conditions. These relationships, and especially the interphase with behavioral and social sciences, are slowly being uncovered. In addition, understanding of the processes that promote aging and how these influence rheumatologic diseases may help identify treatment targets, thus helping in clinical care and decision making unique to older adult populations.

Further, older adults pose unique challenges to the assessment and management of rheumatologic disease. This population often has multimorbidity (defined as ≥ 2 chronic conditions), polypharmacy, frailty, cognitive impairment, and fragmented social support systems.[10–12] Rheumatologic diseases and their clinical manifestations must be understood and managed in the context of these unique challenges and multifactorial pathways that often lead to disability in older adults.[13] This article discusses specific barriers to understanding the biology of aging in rheumatology, and gaps in the assessment, outcomes measurement, and treatment of this unique population. It highlights potential solutions to these barriers and how to bridge the gap so that clinicians can be better prepared to effectively manage older adults with rheumatologic conditions.

GAPS/CHALLENGES IN CURRENT GERIATRIC RHEUMATOLOGY CLINICAL CARE
Gaps in Understanding of the Biology of Aging

Advanced age is a major risk factor for many rheumatologic diseases,[14,15] as it is for many other diseases (eg, atherosclerosis, neurodegenerative disease) but the specific aging-related pathogenic mechanism underlying this association is unclear. Aging is a systemic phenomenon, thus it is conceivable that aging-related diseases of different organ systems may be connected through the same underlying mechanisms. This concept of common aging mechanisms leading to a host of diseases related to aging has led the NIH to initiate and promote geroscience research in an effort to understand the link between aging and aging-related chronic diseases.[9] During the 2013 Geroscience Summit, 7 interconnected processes emerged as potential drivers of the aging process that may govern the pathogenesis of aging-related diseases.[9] A greater understanding of the underlying mechanisms may provide insights into treatment targets for aging-related diseases, including rheumatologic diseases, and ultimately contribute to increasing disease-free life span. The so-called 7 pillars of aging and how they may be associated with rheumatologic diseases in older adults are reviewed here.

Adaptation to stress

Human beings are chronically exposed to stress (physical, social, and psychological), to which neurohumoral, metabolic and immunologic responses are mounted.[16] Chronic stress has been associated with both onset and worse outcomes in rheumatologic diseases. At the level of the individual there exist differences in vulnerability to stressors and responses, with some individuals showing either suboptimal or exaggerated responses.[16] This finding is linked to the question of how age may influence psychological, physiologic, and biological resiliencies. The relationships between stress response, aging pathways, and aging are seen in invertebrate models, but clear evidence from human studies are lacking.[17] Findings regarding the relationship between stress and leukocyte telomere shortness,[18] coupled with the finding that telomere length at birth is affected by prenatal stress,[19] are especially noteworthy because telomere shortening in chondrocytes and leukocytes has been observed in OA.[20,21] Understanding such differences in adaptation to stress, and why some patients may be more resilient than others, may provide key insights into pathogenic mechanisms. Further, identifying biomarkers for the aging process that may help detect vulnerable patients early in the course of the disease, when interventions may be effective, are key areas that merit further research.

Epigenetics

Epigenetics refers to the changes in the genome that do not affect the DNA sequence, and includes DNA methylation, posttranslational histone code, and noncoding RNAs.[9] Aging-related epigenetic changes may influence the rate of aging and are being evaluated in other chronic age-dependent diseases (cancer and Alzheimer disease) using genome-wide association studies.[22] Epigenetic mechanisms have been implicated in the pathogenesis of SLE, RA, scleroderma, and OA.[23] Aging-related epigenetic changes (eg, DNA methylation) have also been linked to abnormal T-cell function that may in turn contribute to the high incidence of autoimmunity in old age.[24] Further, the emergence of evidence for the role of epigenetic drift in RA (which could result in resistance to apoptosis, such as in fibroblastlike synovio-cytes), OA, and other diseases is relevant but warrants more investigation.[23] In addi-tion, the possibility of reversal of aging by targeting epigenetic mechanisms is an promising area of research and may provide novel approaches to the treatment of age-related rheumatologic diseases.[25]

Inflammation or inflammaging

First described by Franceschi and colleagues,[26] so-called inflammaging refers to chronic, low-grade inflammatory response to chronic antigenic burden, implicated in aging-related diseases. Inflammaging is in contrast with acute inflammation, which is an acute immunologic response to injury or other stimuli.[27] Evidence for aging being a proinflammatory state comes from studies in which increased sys-temic levels of proinflammatory cytokines are noted in healthy older adults compared with young adults, as well as in other states of unsuccessful ag-ing.[26,28–30] How chronic inflammation contributes to aging and aging-related dis-eases is unclear, although immune senescence seems to play a role through depletion of immunologic reserve. Cell senescence was initially described by Hay-flick and colleagues[31] as a phenomenon wherein normal cells lose the ability to pro-liferate after multiple cycles of proliferation in in-vitro cell cultures. Senescent cells produce a host of proteins known as senescence-associated secretory phenotypes (SASPs),[32] which contribute to chronic inflammation in aging. One of the key SASP proteins, interleukin-6, has been associated with many rheumatologic diseases, including RA, OA, PMR, and GCA.[33–35] The role of senescent T cells in the patho-genesis of RA has been widely reviewed.[36] Cellular senescence of chondrocytes has also been implicated in OA.[37] However, mechanistic studies showing the role of SASP proteins or inflammaging in the pathogenesis of aging-related rheumato-logic diseases are lacking and merit evaluation. Senolytics, a new class of drugs targeting the removal of senescence cells with the goal of slowing aging and age-related diseases, have been successfully tested in animals.[38] However, the feasibility and effectiveness of this approach in humans and in rheumatologic dis-eases are unclear.

Macromolecular damage/oxidative stress injury

The Harman free radical theory of aging states that oxidative damage to DNA, other cellular components, and tissues accumulates over time and leads to aging, disease, and death.[39,40] A state of oxidative stress occurs when there is macromolecular dam-age of DNA, lipids, or proteins, resulting in imbalance between production of reactive oxygen species/free radicals (chemical species with unpaired electrons) and antioxi-dant defense mechanisms in the body.[41] Support for macromolecular damage and oxidative stress in aging is provided by a study showing decrease in oxidative stress markers and increase in life span with caloric restriction.[42] Although the specific role of oxidative stress injury with aging and aging-related diseases is still under investiga-tion, associations between markers of oxidative stress and aging and aging-related diseases have been reported and summarized in a recent review of published litera-ture.[41,43] Levels of oxidative stress markers were shown to increase with age in a small series of human subjects.[44–46] The aging-associated diseases shown to be associated with oxidative stress markers include Alzheimer disease,[46,47] atherosclerosis/cardio-vascular disease,[48,49] and cancer.[50] Regarding the association of oxidative stress markers and arthritis, epidemiologic studies indicate that agents causing oxidative stress, such as silica, smoking, and infections, are associated with onset and flare of several autoimmune disorders.[51,52] Oxidative damage can cause DNA damage, resulting in autoantigenesis and contributing to the induction of autoimmune diseases such as SLE and RA.[53,54]

Metabolic pathways

Many metabolic processes (eg, glycolysis, fatty acid oxidation, amino acid oxidation, lipogenesis, and ketogenesis) decline with aging. It is unclear whether this decline is a result of aging or a cause of aging. Further, medications targeting metabolic pathways have shown an impact on life span (eg, rifamycin through mammalian target of rapamycin[55] and metformin through activated protein kinase (AMPK)[56]), indicating an intersection of metabolic pathways and aging, with implications for aging-related diseases. An area of interest for rheumatologists and an area of active research is the effect of glucose transporter 1 (GLUT1) on human T-cell growth and proliferation as well as inflammatory response.[57] More research is needed to clarify the role of metabolic pathways in the pathogenesis of aging-related rheumatologic diseases.

Proteostasis

With aging, proteostasis or intracellular protein homeostasis is difficult to maintain and its imbalance is detected in normal aging and in aging-related diseases (Alzheimer or Parkinson disease).[58] Proteostasis pathways are also implicated in inflammation and are of interest in aging-related rheumatologic diseases.[59] The posttranslational protein modifications most observed in diseases, including RA, are glycosylation, citrullination, and carbamylation.[60]

Stem cell regeneration

Some stem cells decline with age but can be rejuvenated by therapy, suggesting that aging is not associated with irreversible loss of stem cells, as shown from aging muscle.[61] This finding has implications for therapy in age-related rheumatologic diseases. Synovial membrane–derived mesenchymal stem cells are detected at higher levels in OA synovial fluid.[62] Because synovial membrane mesenchymal stem cells can develop into multiple cell types,[63] their potential for cartilage regeneration is of interest in aging-related arthritides.

Gaps in Assessment and Outcome Measurement

The evidence base for guiding management, including assessment tools specifically designed for older adults, is limited. Many clinicians use a one-size-fits-all approach to assess and measure outcomes in young and old adults. This approach may not be appropriate because older adults' values, priorities, and expectations regarding treatment may not be the same as for younger populations. Further, it will be increasingly important to incorporate functional outcomes (either performance based on patient-reported) in both clinical care and research for older adults.[64]

Prognostication, goal setting, and time horizons in older adults

As in many fields of medicine, prognostication is an important part of the assessment and development of a treatment plan. This prognostication is particularly important when clinicians need to balance the potential benefits, risks, and cost of chronic therapies (including biologic agents) in the aging rheumatic disease population. Oncology has cancer-specific as well as function-based (eg, Karnofsky Performance Scale) survival prediction tools.[65,66] Similarly, cardiology has developed prognostication tools for cardiac conditions such as congestive heart failure[67] and refractory angina.[68] However, clinicians lack specific tools to help them prognosticate for older adults with rheumatologic conditions. It is important to consider both the absolute and relative risk reduction of a proposed therapy in a frail population that has a limited life expectancy. Until rheumatic disease–specific prognostic tools become available, rheumatologists may consider using disease-agnostic prognostic instruments such as the on-line ePrognosis calculator (http://eprognosis.ucsf.edu/index.php).

With age, questions of prognosis and how aggressively to manage patients are closely linked with individual goals, priorities, and motivations to engage in medical care. Understanding the goals of older patients has direct implications for how clinicians seek to address their rheumatologic conditions. Clinicians are learning that older adults make health-related decisions in different ways than younger adults facing similar health decisions.[69] Research in lifespan development psychology shows how motivations and specific goals vary with age. Motivation affects the degree to which older adults use prior experience, affect, and deliberative skills to make decisions.[69] For example, a growing literature highlights the role of age-related shifts in the ratio of gains and losses. Older adults who face an accumulation of losses of internal and external resources often prioritize maintenance goals and prevention of losses (ie, function). Additional research points to shifting time horizons.[70,71] Older adults frequently view their future time as more limited, and this shift in time horizons may shape motivational priorities and health care decisions. Specifically, older adults often prioritize present-oriented goals to optimize current well-being, focus on positive emotions, and maintain rewarding relationships.[72] As clinicians approach older patients and consider goal setting, they should remember the following quotation: "Don't ask what is the matter with me, ask *what* matters to me."[73,74] To date, little attention has been given to understanding how time horizons, for example, affect the way rheumatologists approach aging patients and navigate conversations about treatment expectations and relevant outcome assessments. Incorporating how older adults are uniquely motivated to change behavior and interact with the health care system has not been systematically evaluated or consistently practiced.

Patient-reported outcomes in older adults

Although various measures have been validated and are widely used throughout the literature, it is debatable whether these instruments fully capture the scope of outcomes that are most meaningful to older populations. In this regard, older adults identify as meaningful the particular consequences of chronic degenerative musculoskeletal pain. In particular, older adults identify the well-established biopsychosocial consequences of chronic pain, including functional, psychological, and social impairments.[75,76,77] Older adults also highlight the adverse impact of pain on fatigue, sleep, and social isolation; consequences that are less commonly assessed in clinical practice.[75] Broadening the assessments from pain to associated functional, psychological, and social outcomes will be important to consider for the aging population.[78,79]

Newer, efficient, state-of-the-science instruments are now available that assess appropriate and relevant domains/outcomes in older adults. Since 2014, the NIH has heavily invested in developing robust patient-centered outcome measures using the Patient-Reported Outcomes Measurement Information System (PROMIS for testing in subpopulations (http://www.nihpromis.org).[80–82] Data collected using PROMIS provide clinicians and researchers with efficient and reliable information about the effect of therapy. How PROMIS instruments may be used in the development and implementation of treatment plans, and used at the point of care to enhance communication, management, and understanding of chronic rheumatologic conditions, is an active area of investigation. Research is underway to evaluate how PROMIS performs in older populations with chronic musculoskeletal pain.[83]

Another critically important area that is fertile for further research is how to assess and evaluate chronic rheumatologic diseases in cognitively impaired older adults.[84]

Joint pain, a common manifestation of rheumatologic diseases, is often assessed by self-report. Presence of dementia and cognitive impairment poses challenges in assessment of pain because of impairment in the ability to report pain, caused by difficulty in recalling and in verbalizing.[85,86] Thus, presence of dementia and cognitive impairment is associated with under-recognition and undertreatment of pain.[87–89] The available behavioral assessment tools, such as Doloplus-2[90] and Pain Assessment Checklist for Seniors with Limited Ability to Communicate (PACSLAC),[91] which rely on nonverbal cues, can be used for the assessment of pain in patients with dementia or cognitive impairment, especially in nursing homes.[92] However, these tools are underdeveloped and have poor psychometric properties.[93]

Gaps in Managing/Treating Older Adults with Rheumatologic Conditions

There is a lack of guidelines that are specific to older adults for most rheumatologic conditions. Older adults are often excluded from clinical trials for various reasons, including multimorbidity, polypharmacy, and fragmented social support systems.[10,11] By not including medically complex older adults in trials, clinicians are unable to fully understand the harm, benefit, and cost ratio of therapies for this specific population. Clinicians often extrapolate clinical decisions from guidelines based on data from younger populations to older patients. This problem is addressed here in the context of multimorbidity, individualized interdisciplinary management, as well as immunizations; all areas critical to consider when treating older adults with rheumatologic conditions.

Multimorbidity and polypharmacy

Given the prevalence of multimorbidity, there has been a push to better understand rheumatologic conditions in the context of coexisting chronic conditions. It is uncommon to care for a patient in rheumatology who has isolated knee OA or RA in the absence of cardiovascular, pulmonary, or renal disease. Although researchers have traditionally avoided the complexity of multiple chronic conditions, it is inevitable that rheumatologists face these each day. For example, the use of nonsteroidal anti-inflammatory medications, which are often better tolerated by young adults, is generally avoided in older adults because of their adverse effects, including increased cardiovascular events and worsening renal impairment. Future research should include heterogeneous populations with multiple chronic conditions in sufficient numbers to measure the benefits and harms of interventions.

Polypharmacy is a direct consequence of multimorbidity. Rheumatologists and geriatricians have to be cognizant of drug interactions as a result of polypharmacy, which makes caring for older adults more complex. Research suggests that the age of the patient influences rheumatologists' decision to escalate care in RA.[94] Future research should consider how ageism plays a role in the quality of care delivered to older adults with rheumatologic diseases. Clinicians also need to carefully consider how, if there is polypharmacy and multimorbidity, escalation or de-escalation of the medication list affects outcomes for this population.

Individualized interdisciplinary management

For older adults with rheumatologic conditions, individualizing the approach to management is critical. Older adults have unique home-life circumstances and divergent abilities to adhere to and sustain management plans. Clinicians must therefore carefully design interventions that are feasible and safe for this population. Developing and implementing individualized plans of care for older adults must be weighed carefully against feasibility, ability to generalize, and cost-effectiveness. Implementing an individualized care plan for an older adult with rheumatologic conditions (among other comorbidities) involves an interdisciplinary team, often including (as available) rheumatologist, geriatrician, physical and/or occupational therapist, psychologist, or behavioral interventionist. As outlined in a review on persistent pain in older adults, combining pharmacologic, nonpharmacologic, and rehabilitative (activity-based) approaches in addition to a strong therapeutic alliance between the patient and physician is essential in setting, adjusting, and achieving realistic goals of therapy.[78]

Immunizations

One area of specific interest in geriatric rheumatology and one that bridges the biology of aging and clinical implications, is vaccine efficacy in later life. Age-related changes in immune function include decline in efficacy of vaccinations in older adults.[95] Based on a review of 31 vaccine antibody response studies conducted from 1986 to 2002, Goodwin and colleagues[95] calculated 7% to 53% efficacy of the influenza vaccine in older adults compared with 70% to 90% in younger adults. These investigators suggested that future research is needed for more immunogenic vaccine formulations specifically for older patients. A recent study found that a high-dose trivalent influenza vaccine, with 4 times as much hemagglutinin, confers superior protection to standard trivalent vaccine.[96] Herpes zoster, reactivation of latent varicella, is more common in older adults and those who are immunocompromised (including patients with inflammatory arthritides and taking disease modifying antirheumatic drugs).[97] The herpes zoster vaccine is recommended for patients with RA who are 50 years of age and older.[98] Additional literature is emerging suggesting that younger adults with autoimmune diseases or inflammatory conditions have rates of herpes zoster that are comparable with or greater than the rates in older adults, and that this population should be considered for vaccination at a younger age cutoff.[99] How this would affect vaccination practices as patients with rheumatologic diseases age is unknown. Further research is needed in older adults with rheumatologic diseases and multimorbidity to determining vaccine efficacy and scheduling. There is tremendous variability in the implementation of guidelines at local levels,[100] and innovative, possibly automated, systems of vaccine delivery by nonphysician providers may be most effective.

BRIDGING THE GAP: A CALL TO ACTION

With aging of the population, there is an urgent need for the workforce to be prepared to manage the rapidly increasing population of older adults with rheumatologic conditions. A recent *New York Times* article highlighted, "Where are the geriatricians?"[101] One potential solution to this shortage is to train subspecialists, including rheumatologists, and other providers in the rheumatology workforce in the appropriate assessment and management of older adults with rheumatologic conditions.

This article discusses the gaps and challenges in the understanding of the biology of aging pertaining to the underlying pathophysiology of age-related rheumatologic diseases, as well as assessment, outcomes measurement, and treatment of rheumatologic diseases in later life. Summarized here are possible ways to bridge the gap, through more research and education, which it is hoped will translate into guidelines that will improve care and foster healthy aging for millions of older adults with rheumatologic diseases.

In the opinions of these authors, and from a research standpoint, the following must be considered:

- Develop aging animal models that are more similar to aging humans for preclinical studies.

- Use age-appropriate animals in evaluating immune-based treatments for rheumatologic diseases that primarily affect older adults.
- Align preclinical models and clinical trial populations, including more appropriate disease phenotype, and ensure that measured outcomes are clinically relevant (ie, outcomes measured in the animal model relate to the human disease).
- Increase the understanding of the relationship between the aging processes and the pathogenesis, clinical manifestation, and treatment of rheumatologic diseases.
- Consider adopting the worldwide strategy of the One Health Initiative: interdisciplinary collaboration and communication between medical and veterinary health care and health research to provide a multidirectional flow of knowledge and synergistic gains for both disciplines.[102]
- Focus research efforts on older adults with multimorbidity and polypharmacy, rather than excluding this medically complex population. Clinical research that involves older adults may benefit from including patient stakeholder input from this group; the group for whom the intervention is intended to benefit. Given the lack of guidelines specific to older adults, now may be a prime opportunity to solicit older adults with rheumatic diseases to participate on guideline panels in order to incorporate their voice and experience.[103]
- Develop novel interventions that can be implemented and disseminated in real-world practice (ie, older adults will have access to the interventions).
- Develop prognostication tools for individual rheumatologic diseases to help guide treatment decisions of these diseases in frail older adults.
- Incorporate functional measures, either performance based or patient reported, in all studies.
- Develop a cadre of future investigators who will serve as opinion leaders in geriatric rheumatology.
  - National Institute on Aging (NIA) has heavily invested in developing research and leadership careers of talented new investigators who are well poised to change theory, practice, and health outcomes related to the health of older adults. The prestigious Beeson award (recently re-named the Paul B. Beeson Emerging Leaders Career Development Award in Aging [K76 NIA mechanism]) serves this purpose.
  - A private/public partnership also exists: the NIA Grants for Early Medical/Surgical Specialists' Transition to Aging Research (GEMSSTAR), which helps early career physicians to establish a track record in aging-related aspects of their specialty.
  - Leverage the Trans-NIH Geroscience Initiative, and increase the participation of, particularly, the National Institute of Arthritis and Musculoskeletal and Skin Diseases (NIAMS) and the National Institute of Allergy and Infectious Diseases (NIAID):
    - Cosponsor conferences and target areas of shared research interests
  - To enhance the pipeline of geriatric rheumatology investigators in academia, pertinent funding opportunities must continue to be provided, perhaps in conjunction with support from foundations (eg, the John A. Hartford Foundation, http://www.jhartfound.org) and organizations (eg, The Atlantic Philanthropies; the Association of Specialty Professors, part of the Alliance for Academic Internal Medicine has a long record of integrating geriatrics within subspecialties) with complementary priorities and shared agendas.
  - The current and next generations of mentors in this field must be cultivated, motivated, and nurtured. A lack of appropriate role models and mentorship

may be one of the primary reasons for talented young investigators leaving academia.[104]

From an education standpoint, the following should be considered:

- Facilitate networking opportunities at national meetings in the form of special interest groups; gathering like-minded individuals helps to drive both research and clinical agendas forward.
- Develop core curricula for geriatric rheumatology that may be disseminated to training programs and that include other professional trainees/providers.
- Develop educational modules that are accessible on-line (eg, via pogo-e, https://www.pogoe.org/about).
- Disseminate research findings to a greater audience/community of clinicians:
  - Peer-reviewed article publication; recent years have seen increased emphasis/focus on aging issues among vulnerable populations.[105]
  - Present research findings at conferences and workshops.
  - Leverage social media forums that provide an avenue to heighten awareness of research findings that are clinically applicable to a geriatric rheumatology population.
  - Partner with advocacy groups and patient stakeholders to make clinical and research voices heard by the community.

As outlined in this article, there is a need to bridge fundamental gaps in research and clinical knowledge to improve the care of older adults with rheumatologic diseases. Clinicians have an important responsibility and opportunity to develop and deliver age-appropriate relevant, effective, and high-value clinical care that will improve outcomes in older adults with rheumatologic disease. By heightening awareness of the intersection of aging with rheumatology it is hoped that the next generation of investigators and clinicians will be inspired to approach their careers and patient care with a commitment to aging.

REFERENCES

1. US Census Bureau. The next four decades: the older population in the United States: 2010 to 2050. In: Vincent GK, Velkoff VA, editors. Washington, DC: US Department of Commerce. Available at: https://http://www.census.gov/prod/2010pubs/p25-1138.pdf. Accessed March 26, 2016.
2. Lawrence RC, Felson DT, Helmick CG, et al. Estimates of the prevalence of arthritis and other rheumatic conditions in the United States. Part II. Arthritis Rheum 2008;58:26–35.
3. Loeser RF. Age-related changes in the musculoskeletal system and the development of osteoarthritis. Clin Geriatr Med 2010;26:371–86.
4. Crowson CS, Matteson EL, Myasoedova E, et al. The lifetime risk of adult-onset rheumatoid arthritis and other inflammatory autoimmune rheumatic diseases. Arthritis Rheum 2011;63:633–9.
5. Arnaud L, Mathian A, Boddaert J, et al. Late-onset systemic lupus erythematosus: epidemiology, diagnosis and treatment. Drugs Aging 2012;29:181–9.
6. Boddaert J, Huong DL, Amoura Z, et al. Late-onset systemic lupus erythematosus: a personal series of 47 patients and pooled analysis of 714 cases in the literature. Medicine (Baltimore) 2004;83:348–59.
7. Lalani S, Pope J, de Leon F, et al. Clinical features and prognosis of late-onset systemic lupus erythematosus: results from the 1000 faces of lupus study. J Rheumatol 2010;37:38–44.

8. Mohan SV, Liao YJ, Kim JW, et al. Giant cell arteritis: immune and vascular aging as disease risk factors. Arthritis Res Ther 2011;13:231.

9. Kennedy BK, Berger SL, Brunet A, et al. Geroscience: linking aging to chronic disease. Cell 2014;159:709–13.

10. Rogers WH, Kazis LE, Miller DR, et al. Comparing the health status of VA and non-VA ambulatory patients: the Veterans' Health and Medical Outcomes Studies. J Ambul Care Manag 2004;27:249–62.

11. Reid MC, Bennett DA, Chen WG, et al. Improving the pharmacologic management of pain in older adults: identifying the research gaps and methods to address them. Pain Med 2011;12:1336–57.

12. Tinetti ME, Fried TR, Boyd CM. Designing health care for the most common chronic condition–multimorbidity. JAMA 2012;307:2493–4.

13. Weiner DK. Introduction to special series: deconstructing chronic low back pain in the older adult: shifting the paradigm from the spine to the person. Pain Med 2015;16:881–5.

14. Michet CJ Jr, Evans JM, Fleming KC, et al. Common rheumatologic diseases in elderly patients. Mayo Clin Proc 1995;70:1205–14.

15. Boots AM, Maier AB, Stinissen P, et al. The influence of ageing on the development and management of rheumatoid arthritis. Nat Rev Rheumatol 2013;9:604–13.

16. Epel ES, Lithgow GJ. Stress biology and aging mechanisms: toward understanding the deep connection between adaptation to stress and longevity. J Gerontol A Biol Sci Med Sci 2014;69(Suppl 1):S10–6.

17. Lithgow GJ, Miller RA. Determination of aging rate by coordinated resistance to multiple forms of stress. In: Guarente LP, Partridge L, Wallace DC, editors. Cold Spring Harbor Monograph Archive, Vol. 51. North America: Cold Spring Harbor Laboratory Press; 2008. p. 427–81.

18. Blackburn EH, Epel ES. Telomeres and adversity: too toxic to ignore. Nature 2012;490:169–71.

19. Price JD, Beauchamp NM, Rahir G, et al. CD8+ dendritic cell-mediated tolerance of autoreactive CD4+ T cells is deficient in NOD mice and can be corrected by blocking CD40L. J Leukoc Biol 2014;95:325–36.

20. Price JS, Waters JG, Darrah C, et al. The role of chondrocyte senescence in osteoarthritis. Aging cell 2002;1:57–65.

21. Zhai G, Aviv A, Hunter DJ, et al. Reduction of leucocyte telomere length in radiographic hand osteoarthritis: a population-based study. Ann Rheum Dis 2006;65:1444–8.

22. Brunet A, Berger SL. Epigenetics of aging and aging-related disease. J Gerontol A Biol Sci Med Sci 2014;69(Suppl 1):S17–20.

23. Gay S, Wilson AG. The emerging role of epigenetics in rheumatic diseases. Rheumatology (Oxford) 2014;53:406–14.

24. Tserel L, Kolde R, Limbach M, et al. Age-related profiling of DNA methylation in CD8+ T cells reveals changes in immune response and transcriptional regulator genes. Sci Rep 2015;5:13107.

25. Gray SG. Perspectives on epigenetic-based immune intervention for rheumatic diseases. Arthritis Res Ther 2013;15:207.

26. Franceschi C, Bonafe M, Valensin S, et al. Inflamm-aging. An evolutionary perspective on immunosenescence. Ann N Y Acad Sci 2000;908:244–54.

27. Freund A, Orjalo AV, Desprez PY, et al. Inflammatory networks during cellular senescence: causes and consequences. Trends Mol Med 2010;16:238–46.

28. Cohen HJ, Pieper CF, Harris T, et al. The association of plasma IL-6 levels with functional disability in community-dwelling elderly. J Gerontol A Biol Sci Med Sci 1997;52:M201–8.
29. Wei J, Xu H, Davies JL, et al. Increase of plasma IL-6 concentration with age in healthy subjects. Life Sci 1992;51:1953–6.
30. Hager K, Machein U, Krieger S, et al. Interleukin-6 and selected plasma proteins in healthy persons of different ages. Neurobiol Aging 1994;15:771–2.
31. Hayflick L, Moorhead PS. The serial cultivation of human diploid cell strains. Exp Cell Res 1961;25:585–621.
32. Coppe JP, Patil CK, Rodier F, et al. Senescence-associated secretory pheno-types reveal cell-nonautonomous functions of oncogenic RAS and the p53 tumor suppressor. PLoS Biol 2008;6:2853–68.
33. Caplanne D, Le Parc JM, Alexandre JA. Interleukin-6 in clinical relapses of poly-myalgia rheumatica and giant cell arteritis. Ann Rheum Dis 1996;55:403–4.
34. Alvarez-Rodriguez L, Lopez-Hoyos M, Mata C, et al. Circulating cytokines in active polymyalgia rheumatica. Ann Rheum Dis 2010;69:263–9.
35. Roche NE, Fulbright JW, Wagner AD, et al. Correlation of interleukin-6 produc-tion and disease activity in polymyalgia rheumatica and giant cell arteritis. Arthritis Rheum 1993;36:1286–94.
36. Weyand CM, Yang Z, Goronzy JJ. T-cell aging in rheumatoid arthritis. Curr Opin Rheumatol 2014;26:93–100.
37. Loeser RF. Aging and osteoarthritis: the role of chondrocyte senescence and aging changes in the cartilage matrix. Osteoarthritis cartilage 2009;17:971–9.
38. Zhu Y, Tchkonia T, Pirtskhalava T, et al. The Achilles' heel of senescent cells: from transcriptome to senolytic drugs. Aging cell 2015;14:644–58.
39. Harman D. Aging: a theory based on free radical and radiation chemistry. J Gerontol 1956;11:298–300.
40. Kirkwood TB. Understanding the odd science of aging. Cell 2005;120:437–47.
41. Richardson AG, Schadt EE. The role of macromolecular damage in aging and age-related disease. J Gerontol A Biol Sci Med Sci 2014;69(Suppl 1):S28–32.
42. Bokov A, Chaudhuri A, Richardson A. The role of oxidative damage and stress in aging. Mech Ageing Dev 2004;125:811–26.
43. Jacob KD, Noren Hooten N, Trzeciak AR, et al. Markers of oxidant stress that are clinically relevant in aging and age-related disease. Mech Ageing Dev 2013; 134:139–57.
44. Humphreys V, Martin RM, Ratcliffe B, et al. Age-related increases in DNA repair and antioxidant protection: a comparison of the Boyd Orr Cohort of elderly sub-jects with a younger population sample. Age Ageing 2007;36:521–6.
45. Trzeciak AR, Mohanty JG, Jacob KD, et al. Oxidative damage to DNA and single strand break repair capacity: relationship to other measures of oxidative stress in a population cohort. Mutat Res 2012;736:93–103.
46. Montine TJ, Peskind ER, Quinn JF, et al. Increased cerebrospinal fluid F2-isoprostanes are associated with aging and latent Alzheimer's disease as iden-tified by biomarkers. Neuromolecular Med 2011;13:37–43.
47. Lovell MA, Gabbita SP, Markesbery WR. Increased DNA oxidation and decreased levels of repair products in Alzheimer's disease ventricular CSF. J Neurochem 1999;72:771–6.
48. Kedziora-Kornatowska K, Czuczejko J, Pawluk H, et al. The markers of oxidative stress and activity of the antioxidant system in the blood of elderly patients with essential arterial hypertension. Cell Mol Biol Lett 2004;9:635–41.

49. Demirbag R, Yilmaz R, Gur M, et al. Lymphocyte DNA damage in patients with acute coronary syndrome and its relationship with severity of acute coronary syndrome. Mutat Res 2005;578:298–307.

50. Muller WU, Bauch T, Stuben G, et al. Radiation sensitivity of lymphocytes from healthy individuals and cancer patients as measured by the comet assay. Radiat Environ Biophys 2001;40:83–9.

51. Miller FW, Alfredsson L, Costenbader KH, et al. Epidemiology of environmental exposures and human autoimmune diseases: findings from a National Institute of Environmental Health Sciences Expert Panel Workshop. J Autoimmun 2012; 39:259–71.

52. Sanz-Cameno P, Medina J, Garcia-Buey L, et al. Enhanced intrahepatic inducible nitric oxide synthase expression and nitrotyrosine accumulation in primary biliary cirrhosis and autoimmune hepatitis. J Hepatol 2002;37:723–9.

53. Perl A. Oxidative stress in the pathology and treatment of systemic lupus erythematosus. Nat Rev Rheumatol 2013;9:674–86.

54. Altindag O, Karakoc M, Kocyigit A, et al. Increased DNA damage and oxidative stress in patients with rheumatoid arthritis. Clin Biochem 2007;40:167–71.

55. Inoki K, Kim J, Guan KL. AMPK and mTOR in cellular energy homeostasis and drug targets. Annu Rev Pharmacol Toxicol 2012;52:381–400.

56. Scarpello JH. Improving survival with metformin: the evidence base today. Diabetes Metab 2003;29:6S36-43.

57. Macintyre AN, Gerriets VA, Nichols AG, et al. The glucose transporter Glut1 is selectively essential for CD4 T cell activation and effector function. Cell Metab 2014;20:61–72.

58. Kaushik S, Cuervo AM. Proteostasis and aging. Nat Med 2015;21:1406–15.

59. Liu-Bryan R, Terkeltaub R. Emerging regulators of the inflammatory process in osteoarthritis. Nat Rev Rheumatol 2015;11:35–44.

60. Mastrangelo A, Colasanti T, Barbati C, et al. The role of posttranslational protein modifications in rheumatological diseases: focus on rheumatoid arthritis. J Immunol Res 2015;2015:712490.

61. Conboy IM, Rando TA. Aging, stem cells and tissue regeneration: lessons from muscle. Cell Cycle 2005;4:407–10.

62. Jones EA, Crawford A, English A, et al. Synovial fluid mesenchymal stem cells in health and early osteoarthritis: detection and functional evaluation at the single-cell level. Arthritis Rheum 2008;58:1731–40.

63. de Sousa EB, Casado PL, Moura Neto V, et al. Synovial fluid and synovial membrane mesenchymal stem cells: latest discoveries and therapeutic perspectives. Stem Cell Res Ther 2014;5:112.

64. Kritchevsky SB, Williamson J. Putting Function First. J Nutrition Health Aging 2014;18:467–8.

65. Mor V, Laliberte L, Morris JN, et al. The Karnofsky performance status scale. An examination of its reliability and validity in a research setting. Cancer 1984;53: 2002–7.

66. Pal SK, Katheria V, Hurria A. Evaluating the older patient with cancer: understanding frailty and the geriatric assessment. CA Cancer J Clin 2010;60:120–32.

67. O'Connor CM, Whellan DJ, Wojdyla D, et al. Factors related to morbidity and mortality in patients with chronic heart failure with systolic dysfunction: the HF-ACTION predictive risk score model. Circ Heart Fail 2012;5:63–71.

68. Povsic TJ, Broderick S, Anstrom KJ, et al. Predictors of long-term clinical endpoints in patients with refractory angina. J Am Heart Assoc 2015;4:e001287.

69. Strough J, de Bruin WB, Peters E. New perspectives for motivating better decisions in older adults. Front Psychol 2015;6:783.
70. Lockenhoff CE, Carstensen LL. Aging, emotion, and health-related decision strategies: motivational manipulations can reduce age differences. Psychol Aging 2007;22:134–46.
71. Lockenhoff CE, Carstensen LL. Decision strategies in health care choices for self and others: older but not younger adults make adjustments for the age of the decision target. J Gerontol B Psychol Sci Soc Sci 2008;63:P106–9.
72. Charles ST, Carstensen LL. Social and emotional aging. Annu Rev Psychol 2010;61:383–409.
73. Reuben DB, Tinetti ME. Goal-oriented patient care–an alternative health outcomes paradigm. N Engl J Med 2012;366:777–9.
74. Bynum JP, Barre L, Reed C, et al. Participation of very old adults in health care decisions. Med Decis Making 2014;34:216–30.
75. Makris UE, Melhado T, Lee SC, et al. Illness representations of restricting back pain: the older person's perspective. Pain Med 2014;15:938–46.
76. Gatchel RJ, McGeary DD, McGeary CA, et al. Interdisciplinary chronic pain management: past, present, and future. Am Psychol 2014;69:119–30.
77. Wilkie R, Blagojevic-Bucknall M, Belcher J, et al. Widespread pain and depression are key modifiable risk factors associated with reduced social participation in older adults: a prospective cohort study in primary care. Medicine 2016;95: e4111.
78. Makris UE, Abrams RC, Gurland B, et al. Management of persistent pain in the older patient: a clinical review. JAMA 2014;312:825–36.
79. Fraenkel L, Falzer P, Fried T, et al. Measuring pain impact versus pain severity using a numeric rating scale. J Gen Intern Med 2012;27:555–60.
80. Amtmann D, Cook KF, Jensen MP, et al. Development of a PROMIS item bank to measure pain interference. Pain 2010;150:173–82.
81. Cella D, Riley W, Stone A, et al. The Patient-Reported Outcomes Measurement Information System (PROMIS) developed and tested its first wave of adult self-reported health outcome item banks: 2005-2008. J Clin Epidemiol 2010;63: 1179–94.
82. Cella D, Yount S, Rothrock N, et al. The Patient-Reported Outcomes Measurement Information System (PROMIS): progress of an NIH roadmap cooperative group during its first two years. Med Care 2007;45:S3–11.
83. Deyo RA, Ramsey K, Buckley DI, et al. Performance of a Patient Reported Outcomes Measurement Information System (PROMIS) short form in older adults with chronic musculoskeletal pain. Pain Med 2016;17:314–24.
84. Hadjistavropoulos T, Herr K, Turk DC, et al. An interdisciplinary expert consensus statement on assessment of pain in older persons. Clin J Pain 2007;23:S1–43.
85. Cole LJ, Farrell MJ, Duff EP, et al. Pain sensitivity and fMRI pain-related brain activity in Alzheimer's disease. Brain 2006;129:2957–65.
86. Gibson SJ, Helme RD. Age-related differences in pain perception and report. Clin Geriatr Med 2001;17:433–56, v-vi.
87. Feldt KS, Ryden MB, Miles S. Treatment of pain in cognitively impaired compared with cognitively intact older patients with hip-fracture. J Am Geriatr Soc 1998;46:1079–85.
88. Nygaard HA, Jarland M. Are nursing home patients with dementia diagnosis at increased risk for inadequate pain treatment? Int J Geriatr Psychiatry 2005;20: 730–7.

89. Morrison RS, Siu AL. A comparison of pain and its treatment in advanced dementia and cognitively intact patients with hip fracture. J pain symptom Manag
2000;19:240–8.

90. Pautex S, Herrmann FR, Michon A, et al. Psychometric properties of the
Doloplus-2 observational pain assessment scale and comparison to self-
assessment in hospitalized elderly. Clin J Pain 2007;23:774–9.

91. Fuchs-Lacelle S, Hadjistavropoulos T. Development and preliminary validation
of the Pain Assessment Checklist for Seniors with Limited Ability to Communicate (PACSLAC). Pain Manag Nurs 2004;5:37–49.

92. Lints-Martindale AC, Hadjistavropoulos T, Barber B, et al. A psychophysical
investigation of the facial action coding system as an index of pain variability
among older adults with and without Alzheimer's disease. Pain Med 2007;8:
678–89.

93. Zwakhalen SM, Hamers JP, Abu-Saad HH, et al. Pain in elderly people with severe dementia: a systematic review of behavioural pain assessment tools. BMC
Geriatr 2006;6:3.

94. Kievit W, van Hulst L, van Riel P, et al. Factors that influence rheumatologists'
decisions to escalate care in rheumatoid arthritis: results from a choice-based
conjoint analysis. Arthritis Care Res 2010;62:842–7.

95. Goodwin K, Viboud C, Simonsen L. Antibody response to influenza vaccination
in the elderly: a quantitative review. Vaccine 2006;24:1159–69.

96. DiazGranados CA, Dunning AJ, Kimmel M, et al. Efficacy of high-dose versus
standard-dose influenza vaccine in older adults. N Engl J Med 2014;371:
635–45.

97. O'Connor KM, Paauw DS. Herpes zoster. Med Clin North Am 2013;97:503–22, ix.

98. Singh JA, Saag KG, Bridges SL Jr, et al. 2015 American College of Rheumatology guideline for the treatment of rheumatoid arthritis. Arthritis Care Res
2016;68:1–25.

99. Yun H, Yang S, Chen L, et al. Risk of herpes zoster in auto-immune and inflammatory diseases: implications for vaccination. Arthritis Rheumatol 2016;68:
2328–37.

100. Papadopoulou D, Sipsas NV. Comparison of national clinical practice guidelines
and recommendations on vaccination of adult patients with autoimmune rheumatic diseases. Rheumatol Int 2014;34:151–63.

101. Hafner K. As population ages, where are the geriatricians? New York Times
2016.

102. Malfait AM, Little CB. On the predictive utility of animal models of osteoarthritis.
Arthritis Res Ther 2015;17:225.

103. Fraenkel L, Miller AS, Clayton K, et al. When patients write the guidelines: patient
panel recommendations for the treatment of rheumatoid arthritis. Arthritis Care
Res 2016;68:26–35.

104. Ogdie A, Shah AA, Makris UE, et al. Barriers to and facilitators of a career as a
physician-scientist among rheumatologists in the US. Arthritis Care Res 2015;
67:1191–201.

105. Pruchno R. Veterans aging. Gerontologist 2016;56:1–4.

Update on Crystal-Induced Arthritides

Hossam El-Zawawy, MD, MS[a,b,*], Brian F. Mandell, MD, PhD[c]

KEYWORDS

- Gout • Geriatrics • Treat to target • Comorbidities

KEY POINTS

- The clinical presentation of gout in the elderly includes more patients with atypical features and offers more of a challenge in clinical differential diagnosis.
- The treatment of gout depends on the stage of the disease as well as the health status and comorbidities of the patient.
- Acute gout attacks are functionally disabling and can lead to a substantial decrease in quality of life. Treatment is aimed at quickly resolving pain and inflammation.
- Definitive curative therapy is to dissolve all of the urate deposits by using urate-lowering therapy; once that is accomplished, attacks will no longer occur.

INTRODUCTION

Microcrystalline disease, predominantly owing to monosodium urate (MSU) deposition (gout) is the most common cause of inflammatory arthritis. The prevalence of clinical gout increases with age in both men and women[1] to approximately 8% in men over the age of 75.[2] This increase occurs for several reasons, to be outlined elsewhere in this article. Gouty arthritis is preceded in patients with hyperuricemia by the clinically silent deposition of MSU in and around intraarticular structures as well as in tendons, bursae, and soft tissues. Deposition of MSU occurs when the serum concentration of urate (SUA) exceeds its solubility which is approximately 6.8 mg/dL. The deposition occurs generally over years, so it is not surprising that older individuals with hyperuricemia (defined as having a SUA >6.8 mg/dL), who have had more time for deposition to occur, are at increased risk to develop gouty arthritis as well as frank tophaceous deposits. The most common reason that SUA levels are increased is the inefficient urate transport from serum into urine and the GI tract via specific transporters under genetic control.

Disclosure Statement: The authors have nothing to disclose.

[a] Charles E. Schmidt College of Medicine, Florida Atlantic University, 777 Glades Road, Boca Raton, FL 33431, USA; [b] Department of Rheumatic and Immunologic Diseases, Cleveland Clinic Florida, 2950 Cleveland Clinic Boulevard, Weston, FL 33331, USA; [c] Department of Rheumatic and Immunologic Disease, Cleveland Clinic Lerner College of Medicine, 9500 Euclid Avenue, A50, Cleveland, OH 44195, USA
* Corresponding author.
E-mail address: elzawah@ccf.org

Clin Geriatr Med 33 (2017) 135–144
http://dx.doi.org/10.1016/j.cger.2016.08.010
0749-0690/17/© 2016 Elsevier Inc. All rights reserved.

Additional contributors to SUA elevations, many of which accompany aging, include obesity, medications (including most diuretics, **Table 1**), decreased glomerular filtration rate, and ingestion of beer (including nonalcoholic) and mineral spirits. Women's SUA levels increase after menopause, because estrogen has a uricosuric effect.[3] Although hyperuricemia and gout are strongly associated with insulin resistance, obstructive sleep apnea, hypertension, and the metabolic syndrome, it seems that the common and perhaps only independent factor required for gout to develop is sustained hyperuricemia to a level greater than 6.8 mg/dL.[4]

Because deposited MSU remains in equilibrium with the SUA, a core principle in treating patients with gout is that maintenance of the SUA significantly below its saturation threshold will ultimately result in the dissolution of the MSU deposits and prevent the occurrence of acute gout attacks. The lower the level that the SUA is maintained, the more rapid the dissolution of the deposits and the sooner the resolution of gout attacks. This principle holds true for young and elderly patients. With usual therapy, the dissolution takes months to years to occur and this needs to be considered when making treatment plans in the very old and others in whom quality of life may dictate need for rapid improvement. The inverse relationship between rate of resolution and SUA level is the basis for why the ultimate target for SUA in those patients with visible/palpable tophi is typically lower (<5.0 mg/dL) than those without tophi (<6.0 mg/dL) because these tophi presumably reflect a higher total urate burden, which in turn will take longer to dissolve. Whatever the final SUA target, orally dosed urate-lowering therapy (ULT) should generally be initiated at a low dose and slowly escalated to the dose necessary to achieve and maintain the desired SUA. Slow escalation should be prescribed to decrease the chance of a "mobilization" attack of gout from the sudden decrease in urate level and to hopefully reduce the likelihood of the patient having an allopurinol hypersensitivity reaction.[5]

Acute gout attacks can be treated successfully with any of several classes of antiinflammatory medications. Corticosteroids, nonsteroidal antiinflammatory drugs (NSAIDs) and interleukin-1 antagonists have been demonstrated in clinical studies to resolve gout attacks. The choice of agent used to treat acute gout is generally dictated by the patient's comorbidities, the potential for adverse interactions with other medications, and personal tolerance of the different antiinflammatory drugs. Older patients often have several of these confounding issues, often making treatment decisions more complicated and limiting therapeutic options.

GOUT PRESENTATION IN THE GERIATRIC POPULATION CAN DIFFER FROM CLASSIC GOUT SEEN IN MIDDLE-AGED MEN

Gout in middle-aged and younger patients classically presents as a recurrent and intermittent disease of the lower extremity of males. The gender difference parallels

Table 1 Drug induced hyperuricemia	
Mechanism	**Drugs**
Increased uric acid production	Cytotoxic chemotherapy, filgrastim, ribavirin/interferon
Reduced renal clearance of uric acid	Angiotensin-converting enzyme inhibitors, cyclosporine, thiazide and loop diuretics, ethambutol, tacrolimus, low-dose aspirin (mild)
Increased urate production and decreased clearance	Niacin

the average serum urate level, which is higher in men. After menopause, women experience an increase in their SUA owing to the loss of the estrogen's uricosuric effect, which can be attenuated by estrogen replacement therapy. For example, in a recent emergency department-based clinical study comparing prednisolone therapy with indomethacin, the average age of enrolled patients was 65 years and 79% were men. Of the participating women in the study, approximately 90% were postmenopausal.[6] As the population ages, the gender disparity of gout narrows, which is related to the delayed onset of hyperuricemia in women. Beyond this observation, there may be other incompletely understood differences between how men and women react to hyperuricemia.

The clinical presentation of gout in the elderly includes more patients with "atypical" features and generally offers more of a diagnostic dilemma. Involvement of joints already damaged by osteoarthritis are seemingly prone to acute gout. This may be owing in part to decreased local solubility of urate as a result of altered proteoglycan composition. Gout attacks in distal finger joints as well as tophus formation at the site of Heberden's nodes of osteoarthritis can be misinterpreted as "inflammatory osteoarthritis" (**Fig. 1**). This pattern has most frequently been described in postmenopausal women on diuretics, but also can occur in men. Some authors have described an increased frequency of polyarticular attacks in older patients.[7,8] If more indolent, then this type of presentation may mimic rheumatoid arthritis or chronic calcium pyrophosphate deposition disease ("pseudogout"). Because bacterial septic arthritis is more common in the elderly, this important consideration must be resolved definitively by synovial fluid analysis and culture. In patients with severe dementia who cannot

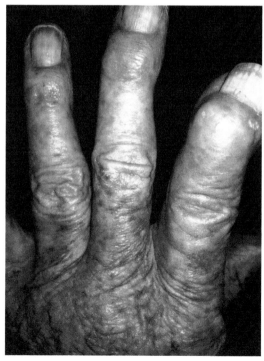

Fig. 1. Tophus on index finger.

clearly articulate their health issues, gout attacks may manifest as fever and/or a further change in cognitive status. Axial involvement with gout has historically been felt to be uncommon, but recent imaging studies indicate that gout can and does involve the spine. Indeed, gout in the spine has been misdiagnosed as compression fracture, metastatic cancer, and infection.[9,10] Unfortunately, these possibilities may not be easily distinguished from tophaceous gout by advanced imaging such as nuclear or MR scanning.

TREATMENT OF GOUT

The treatment of gout depends on the stage of the disease as well as the health status and comorbidities of the patient. Acute attacks need to be diagnosed appropriately and ameliorated promptly to relieve the patient's pain, hopefully without introducing complications related to the therapy. Particularly in patients who have suffered previous attacks of gout, long-term treatment decisions become paramount in importance. Options include (1) treatment with uric acid–lowering agents, which can both dissolve the excess MSU deposits and prevent further gout attacks, (2) treatment with prophylactic low dose antiinflammatory medication, such as daily colchicine to reduce the number and severity of attacks, and (3) watchful waiting, with ad hoc treatment of additional attacks when they occur with high-dose antiinflammatory medications. Each approach has associated risks and benefits.

MANAGEMENT OF ACUTE GOUT ATTACKS

Acute gout attacks are functionally disabling and can lead to a substantial decrease in quality of life. Treatment is aimed at quickly resolving pain and inflammation. In most cases, the choice of the medication will be dictated by the patient's comorbid conditions. There are 4 main groups of medications to treat acute gout attacks: NSAIDs, glucocorticoids (systemic or intraarticular, adrenocorticotrophic hormone), anti–interleukin-1 (eg, anakinra, an interleukin-1 receptor antagonist), and colchicine. It must always be kept in mind that treatment of the acute attacks of gout does not address the primary disease process, which is the abnormal deposition of MSU.

NSAIDs are effective and are the traditional "gold standard" therapy for the treatment of acute gout attacks. All NSAIDs are typically effective when given at full antiinflammatory doses. This includes celecoxib, a cyclooxygenase-2 selective NSAID, although much higher dosing than usual was used in the trial demonstrating its efficacy (1200 mg load on day 1 followed by 400 mg bid as opposed to 200 mg bid).[11] However, NSAID use is potentially associated with a number of adverse reactions, including acute kidney injury, gastric and intestinal ulcers and bleeding, fluid retention, platelet dysfunction, and, less commonly, headache and confusion (particularly with indomethacin). Virtually all of these complications seem to occur more frequently in the elderly. Additionally, several studies suggest a slight increased risk of myocardial infarction or composite cardiovascular adverse outcomes in patients taking NSAIDs, and perhaps cyclooxygenase-2 selective drugs in particular. For these reasons, there has been a trend in many communities for physicians to use alternatives to NSAIDs to treat acute gout attacks, especially in the elderly.

Corticosteroids have been used for years to treat attacks of gout, although there are few clinical trials documenting efficacy. A recent "pragmatic" trial demonstrated equal efficacy of 30 mg/d of prednisolone as for indomethacin in treating acute gout.[6] Although prednisone and other antiinflammatory steroids have many well-recognized severe metabolic and other side effects with chronic use, their short-term use may be safer than that of high-dose NSAIDs in treating acute gout attacks.

Nevertheless, hyperglycemia, sodium/fluid retention, and various degrees of agitation may occur, and patients and their caregivers should be warned regarding these adverse effects. In a study of 13 patients, which included 6 patients (age range, 66–85 years), gout attacks resolved completely within 7 to 10 days using glucocorticoids. The steroid dose was started at 20 to 50 mg and tapered over a mean duration of 10 days.[12] If possible, steroid therapy should be continued in full dose until the attack resolves, and then tapered over several days to off (or back to the baseline dose if the patient was taking a steroid chronically). "Medrol dose packs" (blister packs of a defined dose of a tapering regimen of methylprednisolone pills) can be used to provide simplified instructions. However, sometimes the duration of therapy with dose packs is insufficient and the attack never fully resolves or even rebounds, requiring additional therapy. Intraarticular steroid injections are quite effective and their use limits the potential for systemic side effects. Infection should be excluded and close follow-up of patients receiving intraarticular injection is necessary. Some anatomic locations are difficult to inject, such as the small joints of the fingers and toes and midfoot joints. Intramuscular adrenocorticotrophic hormone is effective, but it is expensive and it has essentially the same metabolic side effects as prednisone. The benefits of steroids in terms of avoiding renal and gastrointestinal complications may be outweighed in some patients by the fluid retention, hyperglycemia, and cognitive effects.

Colchicine has efficacy in relieving the pain and inflammation of acute gout, and low-dose treatment with 3 pills (1.8 mg total) over 24 hours will lessen the pain and signs of inflammation.[13] However, it may not resolve the attack completely, and other analgesic and/or antiinflammatory medications are required frequently. Some patients have learned that they can abort an impending gout attack if they initiate colchicine therapy as soon as they feel a suspicious twinge. But for many, perhaps most, other approaches to resolve the attack may be preferable. That being said, chronic low-dose colchicine (0.6–1.2 mg/d) can be effective for prophylaxis against attacks and, if the patient is taking prophylactic colchicine, the dosage should not be changed in the setting of an acute gout attack.

The primary inflammatory mediator of the acute gout attack is likely interleukin-1; thus, it is not surprising that specific interleukin-1 antagonists are strikingly successful at treating and aborting acute attacks. Several studies now document the impressively favorable and very prompt response of many (not all) patients with acute gout in response to treatment with short courses of daily subcutaneous 100 mg doses of anakinra.[14,15] Anakinra is a short-acting, soluble, interleukin-1 receptor antagonist that has been used successfully in several reports of hospitalized patients, often with comorbidities limiting the therapeutic options or with prior resistance to corticosteroid therapy. Notably, several patients with successful outcomes had serious infections that were being treated concurrently and/or had recently undergone surgery. Anakinra shares none of the short-term metabolic, renal, or cardiovascular complications of NSAIDs or steroids. Unfortunately, this agent is relatively expensive and it does not presently have a US Food and Drug Administration (FDA) indication for use in treating gout. In the general rheumatology community, and for older inpatients with multiple comorbidities, this approach to treating inpatients with gout has growing popularity. Patients with high body mass index may benefit from 200 mg/d instead of 100 mg/d (higher than suggested by the package insert).

Narcotics have variable efficacy in treating the pain of the acute attack and generally should not be relied on as a sole therapy, because it does not address the underlying inflammatory process. This is particularly true in the elderly in whom the risk of falling may be significantly increased by the combination of pain from the gout and the adverse central nervous system effects of the narcotics.

PROPHYLACTIC ANTIINFLAMMATORY THERAPY FOR PATIENTS WITH GOUT

Between attacks, patients may be asymptomatic. Unless the serum urate is lowered, urate will continue to deposit in and around joint structures. Definitive curative therapy consists of dissolution of all urate deposits. However, this may take years of oral ULT. An alternative, quality of life–driven approach is to provide low-dose prophylactic antiinflammatory therapy and only treat attacks as they occur. Low-dose oral colchicine, with appropriate attention to dosing adjustments based on the estimated glomerular filtration rate and potential drug interactions, is generally well-tolerated and reasonably effective in many patients for the purposes of reducing the expected frequency of gout flares. This approach may be limited by the fact that some patients will experience gastrointestinal intolerance with nausea or diarrhea. More serious complications can arise with chronic ingestion, usually in the setting of decreased renal function and/or with decreased colchicine metabolism owing to effects of other drugs. A painful axonal neuropathy and vacuolar myopathy has been well-described,[16] as has multiorgan failure and death. A number of studies have demonstrated pharmacokinetic interactions with colchicine and other drugs, with clarithromycin arguably being the most clinically significant such interaction based on case reports (**Table 2**).[17] Close attention and monitoring of the creatinine kinase and blood counts is warranted if the patient is also taking a statin, ketoconazole, or other drugs that affect the multidrug transporter or the cytochrome P450 system.[18]

In elderly patients with recurrent or tophaceous gout and who are otherwise healthy, ULT should be considered. As ULT is introduced, a seeming paradoxic increase in gout attacks (mobilization attacks) may occur. For this reason, antiinflammatory prophylaxis is generally used for approximately 6 months after initiation of the ULT, and even longer if tophi are detected on physical examination. Colchicine is used most commonly. Drug levels are not routinely available so empiric dosing is usually 0.6 mg 1 to 2 times per day, with attendant dose adjustments in the setting of renal disease. In colchicine-intolerant patients but without relevant comorbidities, low-dose NSAID therapy (ie, naproxen 250 mg bid) may be used to prevent mobilization attacks, generally being coprescribed with gastric protection. Clinical experience with transplant patients suggests that low-dose prednisone may not be as effective as these other prophylactic agents, but sometimes it is the best option.[19]

Table 2 Important drug interactions with Colchicine and allopurinol		
	Drugs That May Interact	**Adverse Effects**
Colchicine	CYP3A4 inhibitors Strong (clarithromycin, ketoconazole, itraconazole) Moderate (diltiazem, verapamil, erythromycin) P-glycoprotein ABCB1 Cyclosporine, ranozaline and verapamil	At higher risk of myotoxicity and neurotoxicity, especially with the strong inhibitors (particularly clarithromycin)
Allopurinol	AZA	Myelosuppression owing to increased AZA metabolites (mercaptopurine)
	Warfarin	May increase anticoagulant effects

Abbreviation: AZA, azathioprine.

URATE-LOWERING THERAPY

Lowering purine intake, following a heart healthy diet, and avoidance of beer or excessive mineral spirit alcohol ingestion is generally recommended for all patients with gout. A recent cross-sectional analysis of nutrition and serum uric acid in 2 Caucasian cohorts of 9734 and 3031 subjects,[20] and an earlier study of 47,150 men, examined the relationship between diet and gout with the SUA.[21] These studies confirmed some long-standing beliefs, namely that consuming meat, seafood, beer, and liquor increases gout risk. Other risk factors identified were consumption of soft drinks sweetened with sugar or fructose, adiposity, hypertension, and diuretic use. In contrast, diets rich in protein, wine, and purine-rich vegetables were not associated with gout flares. Low-fat dairy products may have a protective effect. Weight loss was also found to be protective. Unfortunately, low purine diets are not very palatable, difficult to adhere to, and are minimally effective at best, lowering serum urate by only 1 to 2 mg/dL. Thus, medications are generally required to treat hyperuricemia and reduce the SUA to a target level of less than 6 mg/dL; a target that is, significantly below the estimated urate saturation point in biological fluids of 6.8 mg/dL.

Preventing recurrent gout attacks and tophi formation requires the long-term reduction in the SUA and then maintaining it at below the saturation point. This can be achieved by enhancing renal excretion of uric acid (probenecid, lesinurad, losartan), decreasing urate synthesis (allopurinol and febuxostat), or by converting urate to the more soluble metabolite allantoin through use of uricase. Infused uricase (pegloticase) essentially supplements with an enzyme that is, absent in humans.

The lower the SUA, the more rapidly tophi are resolved and the sooner that gout attacks stop. However, some epidemiologic studies now suggest that patients with sustained low serum urate levels may be at increased risk for (and progress more rapidly with) Parkinson's disease or vascular or nonvascular dementia.[22] The practical implications of these observations are not yet clear, but it may be prudent in those with features of Parkinson's disease or mild cognitive impairment to avoid prolonged hypouricemia. In such patients, low SUA can be attained at the outset of treatment to dramatically decrease the urate burden and stop attacks from happening, but then the SUA can be allowed to drift up closer to the actual saturation point of 6.8 mg/dL.[23] This concern regarding prolonged hypouricemia must be contrasted with a growing body of data indicating that higher SUA levels contribute to the progression of chronic kidney disease,[24] heart failure, and all-cause mortality.

Currently, the use of uricosuric therapy is limited in the United States. Probenecid has been the major medication for this purpose (losartan and fenofibrate have some uricosuric activity). Probenecid has limited popularity owing to a belief that it has relative limited efficacy and to the fact that it may increase the risk for renal stones. In patients with close to normal renal function, who do not excrete significant (more than approximately 800 mg) uric acid daily, who can drink plenty of fluids and can alkalinize their urine, it may be quite efficacious. It can also be used concurrently with a xanthine oxidase inhibitor (eg, allopurinol).

Lesinurad has just been approved by the FDA. It is a potent and fairly specific antagonist of the urate reabsorbing transporter URAT1, and when used as mandated by the FDA label along with a xanthine oxidase inhibitor, it is strikingly effective at reducing the SUA.[25] Nephrolithiasis has not been a problem, but the occurrence of acute kidney injury was noted in clinical trials, especially when allopurinol (or febuxostat) was not used concurrently. These reversible episodes of AKI might be owing to acute urate tubular nephropathy.

Allopurinol (100- and 300-mg tablets) is the most widely used xanthine oxidase inhibitor. Most physicians prescribe no greater than 300 mg/d. However, this dosage has been demonstrated to reduce the serum urate to less than 6 mg/dL in fewer than 30% of patients.[26] Allopurinol has been approved by the FDA for doses up to 800 mg/d. Guidelines from the British Society of Rheumatology advocate a maximum dose of 900 mg/d. It should be noted that these maximum doses are based on limited data, and not on documented toxicity. Slow upward titration, starting with 50 to 100 mg/d at the initiation of therapy, is the commonly recommended regimen. Although gastrointestinal intolerance is a common problem, it is more likely that concern over the rare, but extremely severe, hypersensitivity reaction (approximately 25% mortality), has contributed to its underuse and underdosing, particularly in the setting of chronic kidney disease. This rare complication happens approximately 3 to 9 times in 1000 patients (the higher estimate likely occurring in patients with chronic kidney disease). It has not been demonstrated that reduction of the target dose will decrease the frequency of hypersensitivity, but the initiation at a low dose, with a very slow dose escalation, may reduce the hypersensitivity reaction risk.[5]

Febuxostat (40- and 80-mg tablets) is a newer oral nonpurine selective inhibitor of xanthine oxidase. In the FACT trial (Febuxostat versus Allopurinol Controlled Trial), a 52-week randomized, double-blind study in hyperuricemic patients with gout, serum urate levels were reduced to less than 6.0 mg/dL in more than 50% of patients receiving febuxostat 80 mg or 120 mg once daily, as compared with only 21% of patients receiving a 300-mg fixed dose of allopurinol who were observed to achieve this goal.[27] This does not imply that allopurinol at higher doses would not be equally effective (no allopurinol dose escalation was done in the trial). Indeed, dose escalation of allopurinol is successful in lowering the SUA to a target of less than 6 mg/dL in almost all patients.[28]

Because allopurinol and febuxostat are not similar in chemical structure, febuxostat is an attractive alternative in patients allergic to allopurinol. This has been studied in a limited number of patients. In 12 of 13 patients with gout (92%) with previously documented severe allopurinol adverse effect, the use of febuxostat was safe.[29] Febuxostat remains far more expensive in the United States than allopurinol. Lesinurad (or probenecid) can be added to either of these medications to significantly improve their efficacy. But even with the combination of a uricosuric and a xanthine oxidase inhibitor it may be difficult to profoundly lower the SUA in select individuals.

Uricase metabolizes urate to the more soluble molecule allantoin, which is excreted readily in the urine. Humans (and great apes) evolutionarily deactivated uricase centuries ago, and thus have higher SUA than most other species. Pegloticase is a recombinant polyethylene glycol conjugated uricase that is FDA approved for intravenous therapy for gout in patients who have failed other ULT. It rapidly and profoundly reduces serum urate to less than 0.5 mg/dL in the majority of patients and can lead to resolution of tophi over months.[30] A predictable side effect of rapidly and dramatically reducing SUA is the occurrence of severe gout flares, despite using prophylactic therapy. Pegloticase is administered by intravenous infusion every 2 weeks; this can be decreased to every 3 weeks in many responder patients. However, most patients develop some antimedication antibodies, most to the polyethylene glycol "coating." Those patients with high titer antibody levels rapidly become drug resistant and experience the overwhelming majority of the infusion reactions, which are usually mild.[31] By checking the SUA before each infusion, most infusion reactions can be predicted and prevented. In essence, discontinuing therapy when a diminished hypouricemic response to the drug is noted is the recommended strategy. Patients who develop high titer drug antibodies and clear the drug from the circulation rapidly are also the patients who experience allergic reactions, despite receiving steroid and antihistamine pretreatment. In the remaining patients who experience an ongoing dramatic lowering of SUA, therapy can be continued until visible tophi are resolved and attacks cease. At that point (or even before) the pegloticase can be stopped and the patient switched back to an oral agent targeting the SUA to a level approximately 6 mg/dL.

SUMMARY

Gout is a chronic disease of deposition of MSU in multiple anatomic locations. Although the major attributed manifestation is the acute gout flare, which must be treated promptly, ideal long-term management requires dissolution of the urate deposition by lowering the serum urate to less than 6.0 mg/dL to ultimately stop flares and prevent the development of a chronic arthropathy and likely worsening/progression of other urate associated metabolic conditions including chronic kidney disease. The decisions surrounding the initiation or intensification of ULT must be individualized, especially in elderly patients. The decision process must include evaluation of the patient's life expectancy, frequency and impact of gout flares, daily function, comorbidities, baseline medications, and the ability to tolerate ULT, gout flare prophylaxis, and the treatment of the acute flares.

REFERENCES

1. Zhu Y, Pandya BJ, Choi HK. Prevalence of gout and hyperuricemia in the US general population: the National Health and Nutrition Examination Survey 2007-2008. Arthritis Rheum 2011;63:3136–41.
2. Mikuls TR, Farrar JT, Bilker WB, et al. Suboptimal physician adherence to quality indicators for the management of gout and Rheumatology asymptomatic hyperuricemia: results from the UK General Practice Research Database (GPRD). Rheumatology (Oxford) 2005;44(8):1038–42.
3. Nicholls A, Snaith ML, Scott JT. Effect of oestrogen therapy on plasma and urinary levels of uric acid. Br Med J 1973;1:449–51.
4. Duskin-Bitan H, Cohen E, Goldberg E, et al. The degree of asymptomatic hyperuricemia and the risk of gout. A retrospective analysis of a large cohort. Clin Rheumatol 2014;33:549–53.
5. Stamp LK, O'Donnell JL, Zhang M, et al. Using allopurinol above the dose based on creatinine clearance is effective and safe in patients with chronic gout, including those with renal impairment. Arthritis Rheum 2011;63(2):412–21.
6. Rainer TH, Cheng CH, Janssens HJEM, et al. Oral prednisolone in the treatment of acute gout. Ann Intern Med 2016;164:464–71.
7. Fam AG. Gout in the elderly. Clinical presentation and treatment. Drugs Aging 1998;13:229–43.
8. Meyers OL, Monteagudo FSE. A comparison of gout in men and women: a 10-year experience. S Afr Med J 1986;70:721–3.
9. Saketkoo LA, Robertson HJ, Dyer HR, et al. Axial gouty arthropathy. Am J Med Sci 2009;338:140–6.
10. Konatalapalli RM, Lumezanu E, Jelinek JS, et al. Correlates of axial gout: a cross-sectional study. J Rheumatol 2012;39:1445–9.
11. Schumacher HR, Berger MF, Li-Yu J, et al. Efficacy and tolerability of celecoxib in the treatment of acute gouty arthritis: a randomized controlled trial. J Rheumatol 2012;39:1859–66.
12. Groff GD, Franck WA, Raddatz DA. Systemic steroid therapy for acute gout: a clinical trial and review of the literature. Semin Arthritis Rheum 1990;19:329–36.

13. Terkeltaub RA, Furst DE, Bennett K, et al. High versus low dosing of oral colchicine for early acute gout flare: twenty-four-hour outcome of the first multicenter, randomized, double-blind, placebo controlled, parallel-group, dose-comparison colchicine study. Arthritis Rheum 2010;62:1060–8.

14. Ghosh P, Cho M, Rawat G, et al. Treatment of acute gouty arthritis in complex hospitalized patients with anakinra. Arthritis Care Res 2013;65(8):1381–4.

15. Thueringer JT, Doll NK, Gertner E. Anakinra for the treatment of acute severe gout in critically ill patients. Semin Arthritis Rheum 2015;45(1):81–5.

16. Kuncl RW, Duncan G, Watson D, et al. Colchicine myopathy and neuropathy. N Engl J Med 1987;316:1562–8.

17. Hung IF, Wu AK, Cheng VC, et al. Fatal interaction between clarithromycin and colchicine in patients with renal insufficiency: a retrospective study. Clin Infect Dis 2005;41:291–300.

18. Terkeltaub RA, Furst DE, DiGiacinto JL, et al. Novel evidence based colchicine dose reduction algorithm to predict and prevent colchicine toxicity in the presence of cytochrome P450 3A4/P glycoprotein inhibitors. Arthritis Rheum 2011; 63:2226–37.

19. Clive DM. Renal transplant-associated hyperuricemia and gout. J Am Soc Nephrol 2000;11:974–9.

20. Zykova SN, Storhaug HM, Toft I. Cross-sectional analysis of nutrition and serum uric acid in two Caucasian cohorts: The AusDiab Study and the Tromsø study. Nutr J 2015;14:49.

21. Choi HK, Atkinson K, Karlson EW, et al. Purine-rich foods, dairy and protein intake, and the risk of gout in men. N Engl J Med 2004;350:1093–103.

22. Hong JY, Lan TY, Tang GJ, et al. Gout and the risk of dementia: a nationwide population-based cohort study. Arthritis Res Ther 2015;17:139–46.

23. Perez-Ruiz F, Herrero-Beites AM, Carmona L. A two staged approach to the treatment of hyperuricemia in gout: the "dirty dish" hypothesis. Arthritis Rheum 2011; 63:4002–6.

24. Levy G, Cheetham TC. Is it time to start treating asymptomatic hyperuricemia? Am J Kidney Dis 2015;66:933–5.

25. Hoy S. Lesinurad: first global approval. Drugs 2016;76:509–16.

26. Perez-Ruiz F, Alonso-Ruiz A, Calabozo M, et al. Efficacy of allopurinol and benzbromarone for the control of hyperuricaemia. A pathogenic approach to the treatment of primary chronic gout. Ann Rheum Dis 1998;57:545–9.

27. Becker MA, Schumacher HR Jr, Wortmann RL, et al. Febuxostat compared with allopurinol in patients with hyperuricemia and gout. N Engl J Med 2005;353: 2450–61.

28. Reinders MK, Haagsma C, Jansen TL, et al. A randomised controlled trial on the efficacy and tolerability with dose escalation of allopurinol 300–600 mg/day versus benzbromarone 100–200 mg/day in patients with gout. Ann Rheum Dis 2009;68:892–7.

29. Chohan S. Safety and efficacy of febuxostat treatment in subjects with gout and severe allopurinol adverse reactions. J Rheumatol 2011;38(9):1957–9.

30. Baraf H, Becker M, Gutierrez-Urena S, et al. Tophus burden reduction with pegloticase: results from phase 3 randomized trials and open-label extension in patients with chronic gout refractory to conventional therapy. Arthritis Res Ther 2013;15:R137.

31. Lipsky P, Calabrese L, Kavanaugh A, et al. Pegloticase immunogenicity: the relationship between efficacy and antibody development in patients treated for refractory chronic gout. Arthritis Res Ther 2014;16:R60.

Index

Note: Page numbers of article titles are in **boldface** type.

A

Abaloparatide, in osteoporosis, 36
Acetaminophen, in osteoarthritis, 47
Acupuncture/dry needling, in rheumatic disorders, 67
Age bias, in prescription of treatment, 3
Aging, as heterogenous process, 61–62
    gaps in assessment and outcome measurement, 123–125
Aging research, gaps in, as applies to rheumatologic clinical care, **119–133**
Alendronate, in osteoporosis, 31, 35
Allopurinol, drug interactions with, 140
    in gout, 142
Anakinra, in gout, 140
Anti-inflammatory agents, nonsteroidal, in osteoarthritis, 47
    topical, nonsteroidal, in osteoarthritis, 44
Anti-inflammatory therapy, prophylactic, in gout, 140
Antirheumatic drugs, oral disease-modifying, 2
Arthritides, crystal-induced, **135–144**
Arthritis, inflammatory, microcrystalline disease as cause of, 135
    rheumatoid. See *Rheumatoid arthritis.*
Atherosclerosis, burden of, at diagnosis of rheumatoid arthritis, 110
    exposures to, as risk factor for rheumatoid arthritis, 109–110
Autoimmune disorders, malignancy and, 73

B

Bisphosphonates, adverse effects of, 33–34
    in osteoporosis, 31, 33–36
Bone mass, effect of bisphosphonates on, 34
Brightness mode (B-mode) US, 55–56, 57, 58
Bursae disorders, 58–59

C

Cachexia, 22
Canale-Smith stiff-person syndrome, and malignancy, 81
Capsaicin, in osteoarthritis, 45
Cardiovascular disease(s), in rheunatoid arthritis, incidence rate among women, 106, 107
    increased in rheumatoid arthritis, 106
    inflammation in, leading to heart failure, 110–111
    risk factors for, in rheumatoid arthritis, 106, 108
        rheumatoid arthritis-specific, 111
    risk in rheumatoid arthritis, role of dyslipidemia in, 108–112

Clin Geriatr Med 33 (2017) 145–151
http://dx.doi.org/10.1016/S0749-0690(16)30106-9
0749-0690/17

geriatric.theclinics.com

Moving?

Make sure your subscription moves with you!

To notify us of your new address, find your **Clinics Account Number** (located on your mailing label above your name), and contact customer service at:

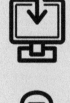

Email: journalscustomerservice-usa@elsevier.com

800-654-2452 (subscribers in the U.S. & Canada)
314-447-8871 (subscribers outside of the U.S. & Canada)

Fax number: 314-447-8029

Elsevier Health Sciences Division
Subscription Customer Service
3251 Riverport Lane
Maryland Heights, MO 63043

*To ensure uninterrupted delivery of your subscription, please notify us at least 4 weeks in advance of move.